THE
joy*of*sex

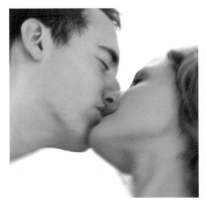

Alex Comfort, M.B., D.Sc.
Susan Quilliam

Three Rivers Press
New York

contents

sauces and pickles 211

preface by Alex Comfort

I am a physician and human biologist for whom the natural history of human sexuality is of as much interest as the rest of human natural history. As with the rest of human natural history, I had notes on it. My wife encouraged me to bring biology into medicine, and my old medical school had no decent textbook to teach a human sexuality course.

Joy was compiled and, very importantly, illustrated, just after the end of that daft and extraordinary non-statute in Western society, the Sexual Official Secrets Act. For at least two hundred years, the description, and above all the depiction, of this most familiar and domestic group of activities, and of almost everything associated with them, had been classified. When, in the sixteenth century, Giulio Romano engraved his weightily classical pictures showing sixteen ways of making love, and Aretino wrote poems to go with them, a leading ecclesiastic opined that the artist deserved to be crucified. The public, apparently, thought otherwise ("Why," said Aretino, "should we not look upon that which pleases us most?") and *Aretin's Postures* have circulated surreptitiously ever since, but even in 1950s Britain pubic hair had to be airbrushed out to provide a smooth and featureless surface.

People today, who never experienced the freeze on sexual information, won't appreciate the propositions of the transformation when it ended – it was like ripping down the Iron Curtain. My immediate predecessor in writing about domestic sex, Dr. Eustace Chesser, was (unsuccessfully) prosecuted for his low-key, unillustrated book *Love Without Fear*, and even in 1972 there was still some remaining doubt about whether *Joy* would be banned by the Thought Police.

The main aim of "sexual bibliotherapy" (writing books like this one) was to undo some of the mischief caused by the guilt, misinformation, and lack of information. That kind of reassurance is still needed. I have asked various people – chiefly older couples – whether *The Joy of Sex* told them things they didn't know, or reassured them about things they knew and already did or would like to do. I have had both answers. One can now read books and see pictures devoted to sexual behavior almost without limitation in democratic countries, but it takes more than a few decades and a turnover of generations to undo centuries of misinformation; and of this material, much is anxious or hostile or over the top. People who worried, when the book first came out, if they did some of the things described in it may now worry if they don't do all of them. That we can't help, nor the fact that the same people who went to doctors because of sexual fear and inhibition under the old dispensation now go complaining of sexual indigestion under the new.

Sexual behavior probably changes remarkably little over the years — sexual revolutions and moral backlashes chiefly affect the degree of frankness or reticence about what people do in private; the main contributor to any sexual revolution in our own time, insofar as it affects behavior, has not been frankness but the advent of reliable contraception, which makes it possible to separate the reproductive and recreational uses of sexuality. Where unanxious books dealing as accurately as possible with the range of sexual behaviors are most valuable is in encouraging the sexually active reader — who both wants to enjoy sex and to be responsible about it — and in aiding the helping professions to avoid causing problems to their clients. It is only recently, as ethology has replaced psychoanalytic theory, that counselors have come to realize that sex, besides being a serious interpersonal matter, is a deeply rewarding form of play. Children are not encouraged to be embarrassed about their play; adults often have been and are still. So long as play is not hostile, cruel, unhappy, or limiting, they need not be.

One of the most important uses of play is in expressing a healthy awareness of sexual equality. This involves letting both sexes take turns in controlling the game; sex is no longer what men do to women and women are supposed to enjoy. Sexual interaction is sometimes a loving fusion, sometimes a situation where each is a "sex object" — maturity in sexual relationships involves balancing, rather than denying, the personal and impersonal aspects of arousal. Both are essential and built-in to humans. For anyone who is short on either of these elements, play is the way to learn: men learn to stop domineering and trying to perform; women discover that they can take control in the give-and-take of the game rather than by nay-saying. If they achieve this, Man and Woman are one another's best friends in the very sparks they strike from one another.

This book has changed considerably since its first edition and it will be revised again in the future as knowledge increases. What will not change is the central importance of unanxious, responsible, and happy sexuality in the lives of normal people. For what they need — in a culture that does not learn skills and comparisons in this area of living by watching — is accurate and unbothered information. The availability of this, and public resistance to the minority of disturbed people who for so long limited it, is an excellent test of the degree of liberty and concern in a society, reflected in the now-old injunction to make love, not war. It is a socially relevant test today.

Alex Comfort, M.B., D.Sc., 1991

preface by Susan Quilliam

I am a relationships psychologist and sexologist whose lifetime aim, through a variety of expert roles, has been to help people enhance their emotional and sexual partnerships. So when the publishers of *The Joy of Sex* approached me to "reinvent" the book for the twenty-first century, it seemed to me the fulfillment of everything I have been working for.

I well remember the original publication of *Joy*, and the awed giggles with which I and my friends read, discussed, and then put into practice its suggestions. So I know firsthand what over the decades proved to be true: *Joy* is an astonishing and inspirational child of its age, born not only out of social but also political changes that irreversibly altered the sexual landscape for individuals, couples, and society. Barely a decade before the book's 1972 publication, the contraceptive pill had, for the first time in history, enabled women to have control over their own fertility. In its wake came increased female education, emancipation, and self-belief, as well as a whole host of liberalizations, sexual and social — increasing permissiveness, more frequent cohabitation, easier divorce, more available erotica, and gay rights.

Joy was not only a product of this revolution, it also helped create it. Dr. Alex Comfort's aim was to write the first book that gave readers accurate knowledge about sexuality, and permission to use that knowledge. The text and illustrations were designed to both reassure the reader that their sexuality was normal and to offer further possibilities with which to expand their sexual menu. He was hugely effective in his intention — 8.5 million copies of *The Joy of Sex* have been sold to date and it has been translated into fourteen languages. More than that, it was a key influence on the social changes of the late twentieth century and has been a byword for sexual vision ever since.

Why, then, reinvent? There have already been content revisions, in the author's lifetime and after his death in 2000, the most recent being the highly successful thirtieth-anniversary edition by Alex's son Nicholas Comfort. But the very changes that *Joy* itself wrought in society have meant that the book has come to need updating in a more fundamental way. This was my task — to re-create *The Joy of Sex* for the contemporary world; to do what Alex Comfort would have done had he been writing today.

The majority of the text remains the same, but substantial additions have been made. Many of these are informational; there have been countless key scientific discoveries in recent years in the fields of physiology, psychology, psychotherapy, and medicine, while the advent of sexology — the specialist study of sexual matters — has resulted in both rigorous academic research and a more widespread public awareness of, and skill in, sex.

8

Alongside these informational updates, a great deal of refocusing has been necessary to reflect social shifts. An intimate relationship is a very different animal from what it was in 1972. It's now largely expected that sex will be part of every love partnership, that bedroom activity will include practices previously considered outrageous, and that these practices will be informed and often suggested via a new raft of technological advances. It's acknowledged that a woman can lead just as much as a man, both in bed and out of it — one reason why the publisher chose a woman to reinvent the book. And it is, albeit slowly, now acknowledged that a couple's sex life lasts well into their later years and increases, rather than decreases, in quality.

Yet along with all these positive developments has come a flurry of problems that weren't predicted in the heady days of 1972. Pressure to have sex; regret that one has had sex; worry that one isn't sufficiently beautiful to deserve sex; worry that one isn't having enough sex or enough good sex. And all that is set beside high rates of pregnancy, abortion, and sexually transmitted infections. In the twenty-first century, as we hastily adapt to a society arguably more sexualized than any previous one, it's a wild world out there.

All of which is why the many changes made to *Joy* have been underpinned by what remains the same — an absolute yet pragmatic optimism around sexuality and its place in our lives. Running throughout the original book was a rock-solid seam of positivity that sex is a good thing and that mature adults, given the right information and inspiration, can be trusted to treat it as such. Despite the headlines and scare stories, I still deeply believe in what Alex Comfort proposed — that sex should be and can be a total joy.

I have loved reinventing the book because Alex Comfort's values and aims are also mine. I too want to present knowledge in an accessible form. To encourage mature decision-making and offer the skills and strategies to do it. To protest attempts to enforce inhibitions on human sexuality. To see sex as the ultimate in human play, but at the same time a developmental essential that helps us grow as people and partners. Above all, to give people not just the technicalities, the fripperies, or the "junk food" of sexual literature, but an intelligent, thoughtful, and "gourmet" treatment of the topic.

In the end I return to, and repeat in my own voice, Alex Comfort's words from his first preface. My intention and my hope is that this book will "benefit . . . the ordinary, sexually active reader — eager to both enjoy sexuality and to be tender and responsible with it." True in 1972. Just as true today.

Susan Quilliam, 2008

i like my body when it is with your
body. It is so quite new a thing.
Muscles better and nerves more.
i like your body. i like what it does,
i like its hows. i like to feel the spine
of your body and its bones, and the trembling
-firm-smooth ness and which i will
again and again and again
kiss, i like kissing this and that of you,
i like, slowly stroking the, shocking fuzz
of your electric fur, and what-is-it comes
over parting flesh. . . . And eyes big love-crumbs,

and possibly i like the thrill

of under me you so quite new

e. e. cummings

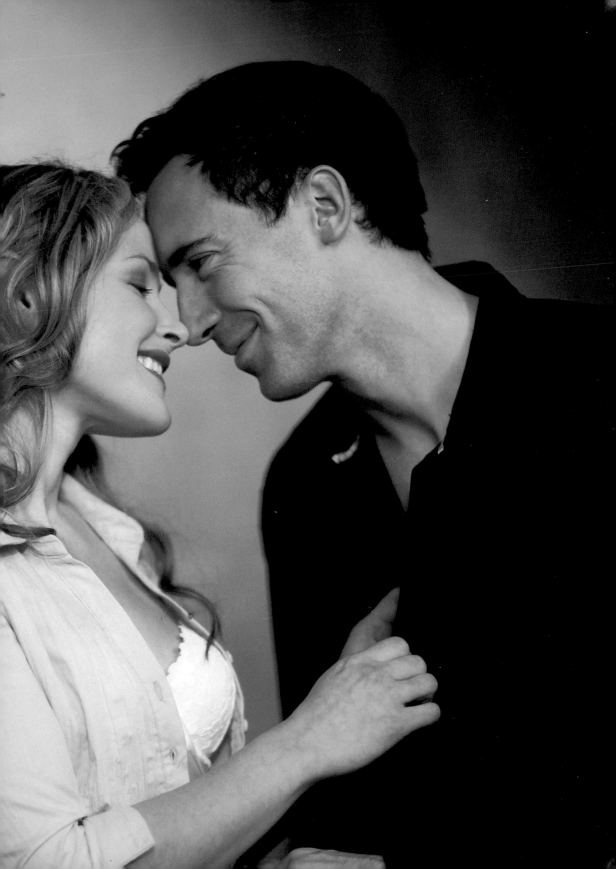

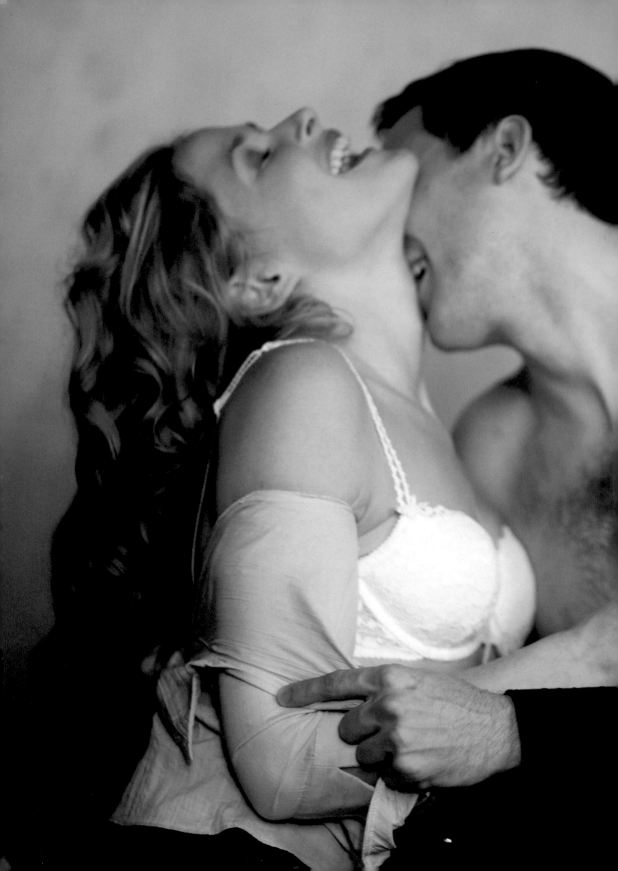

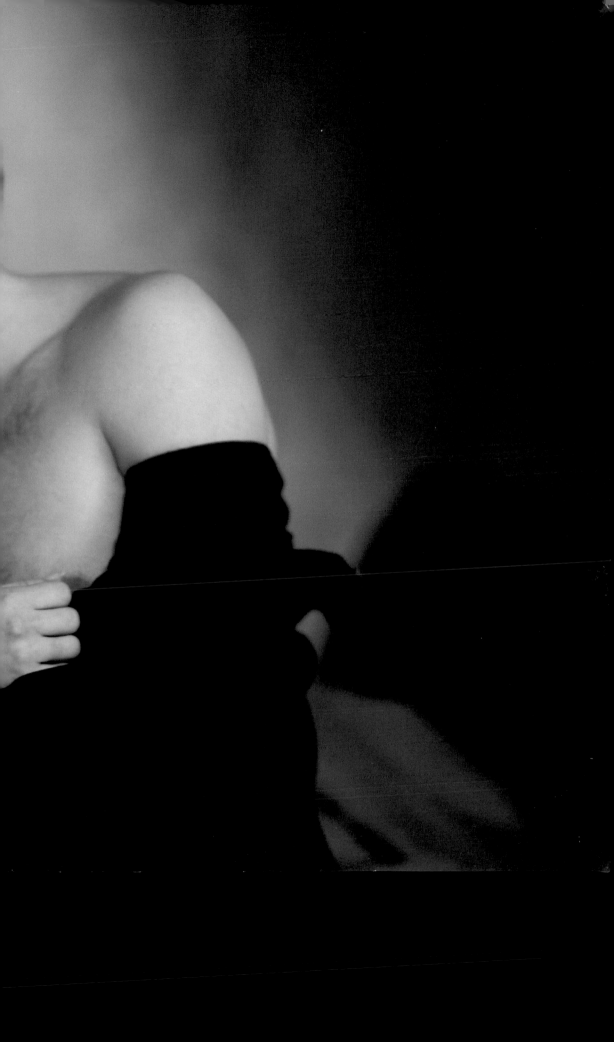

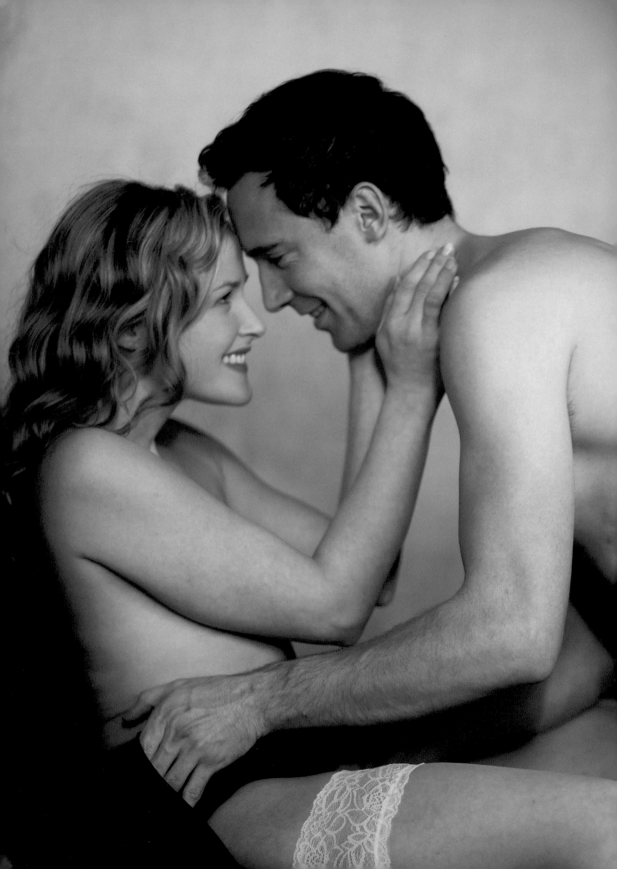

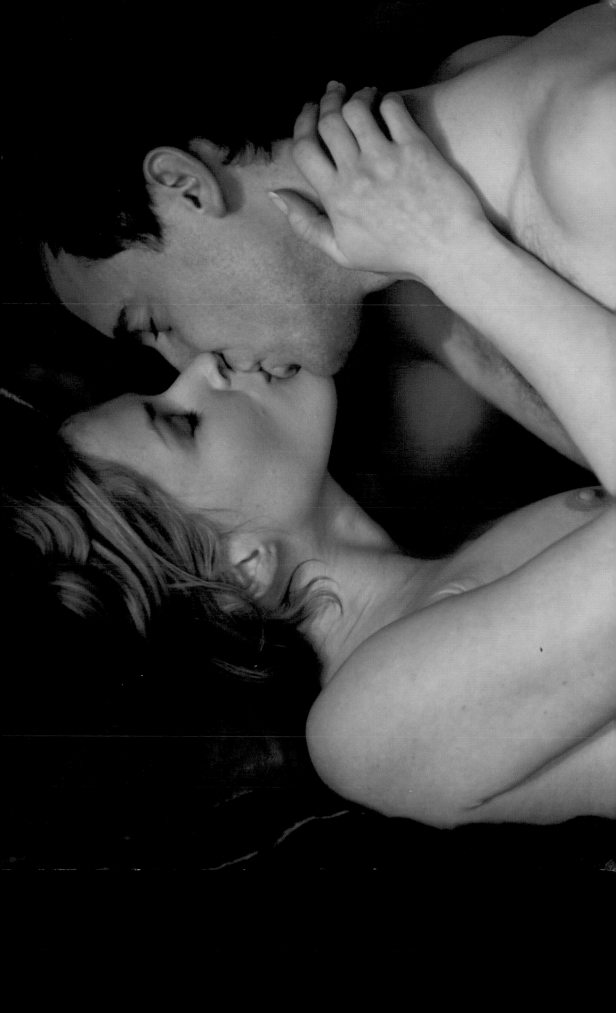

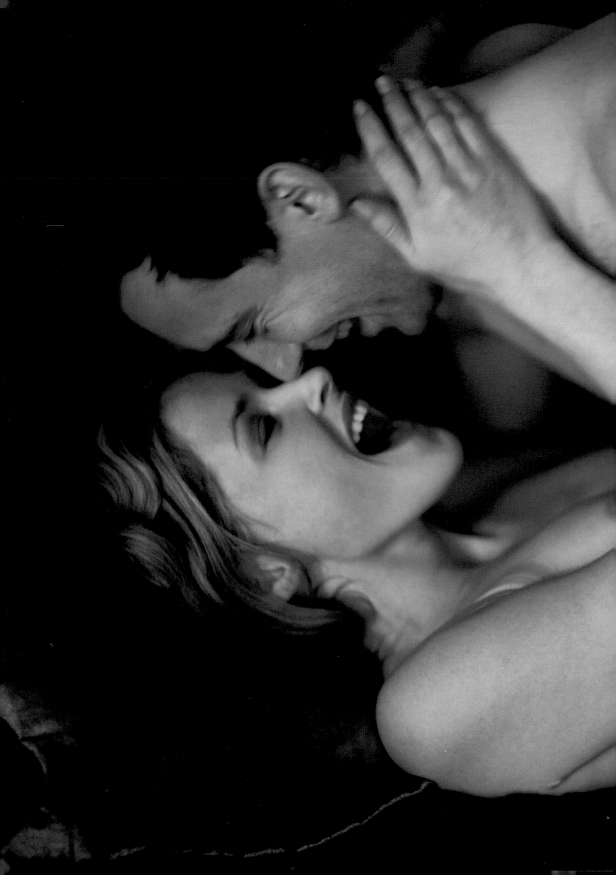

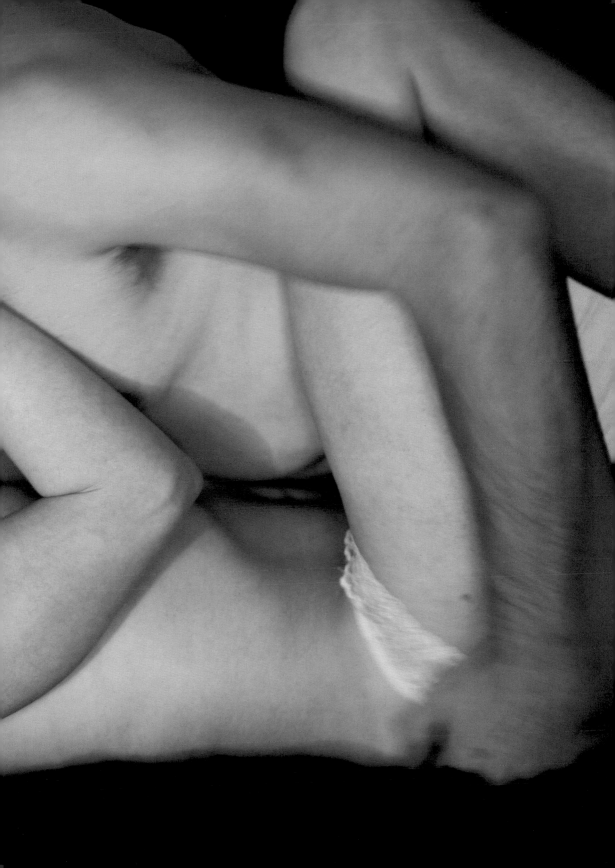

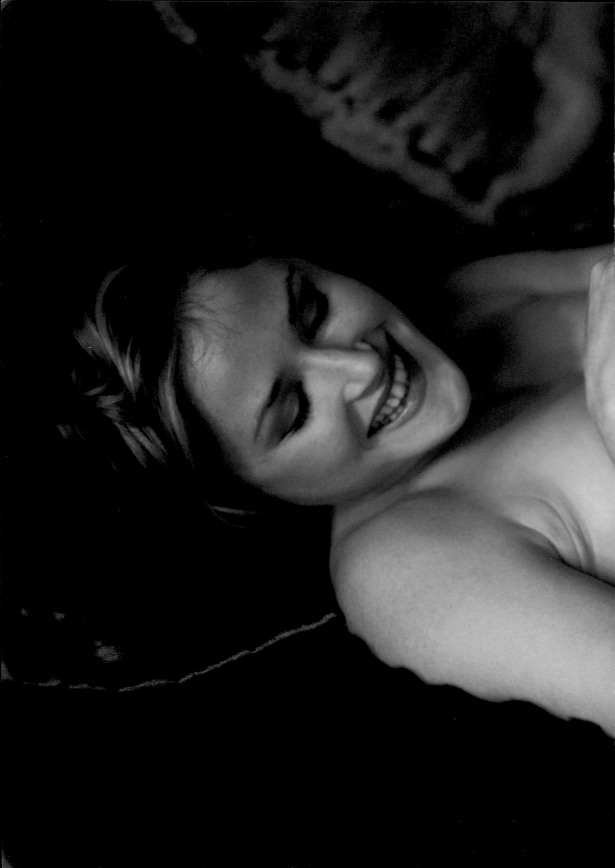

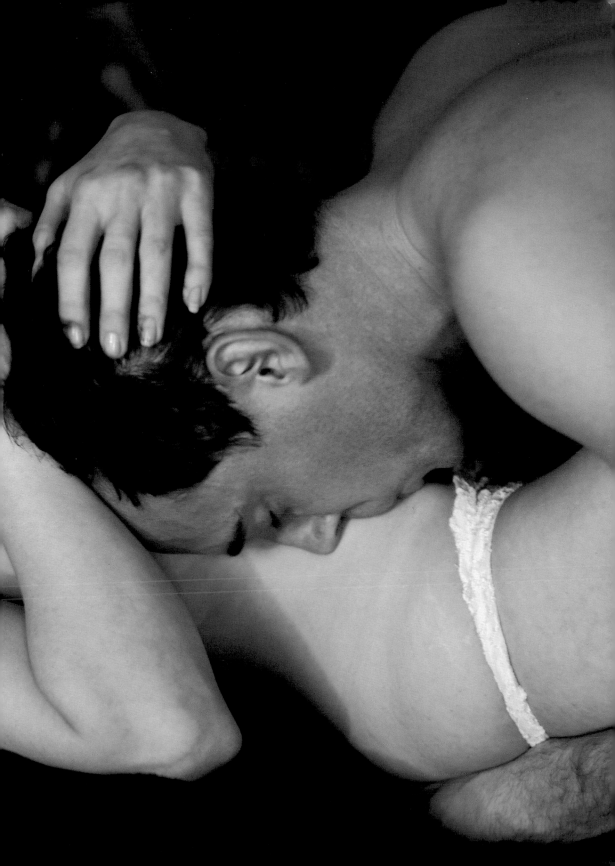

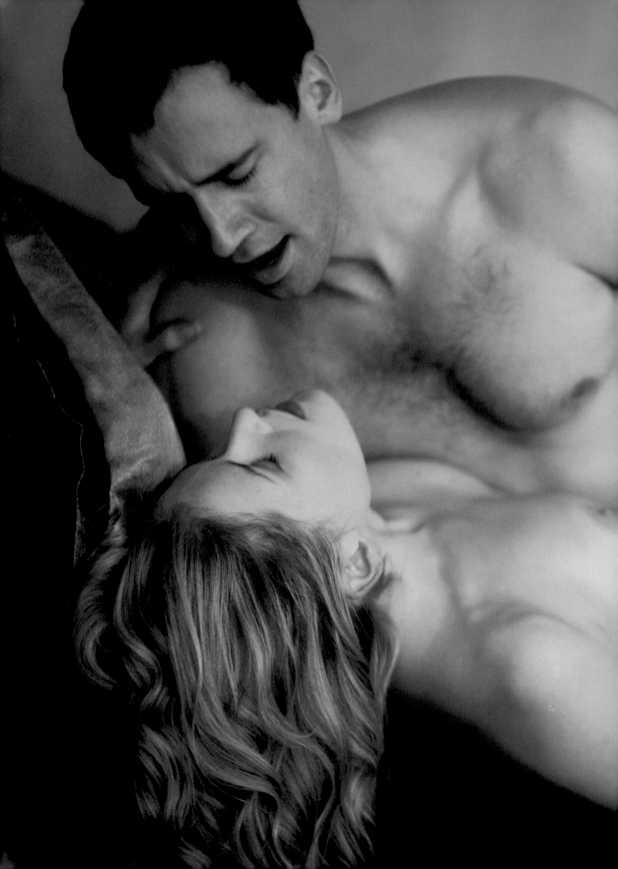

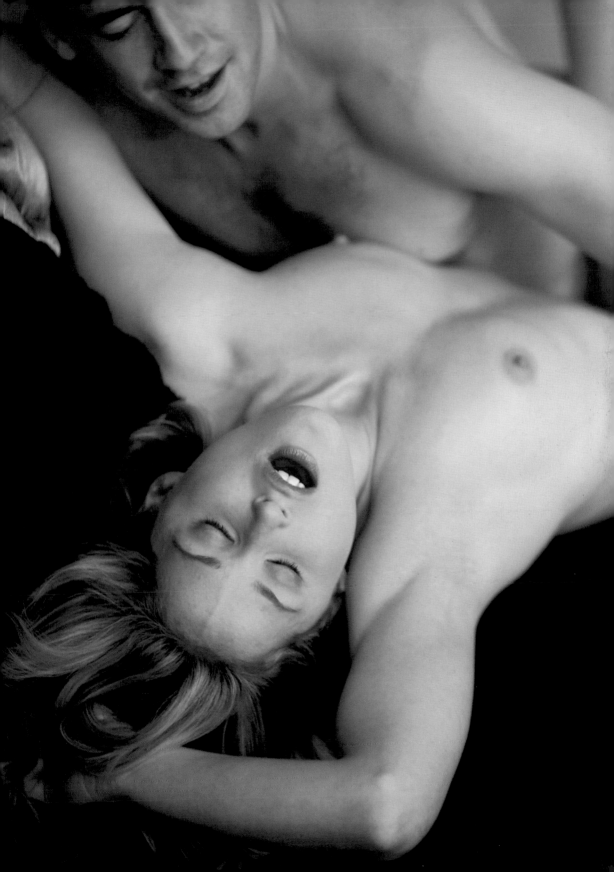

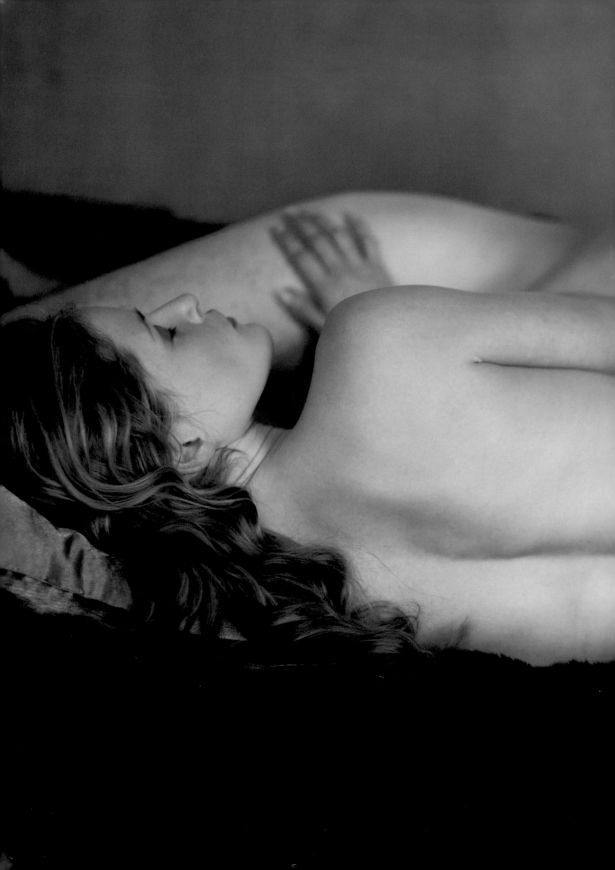

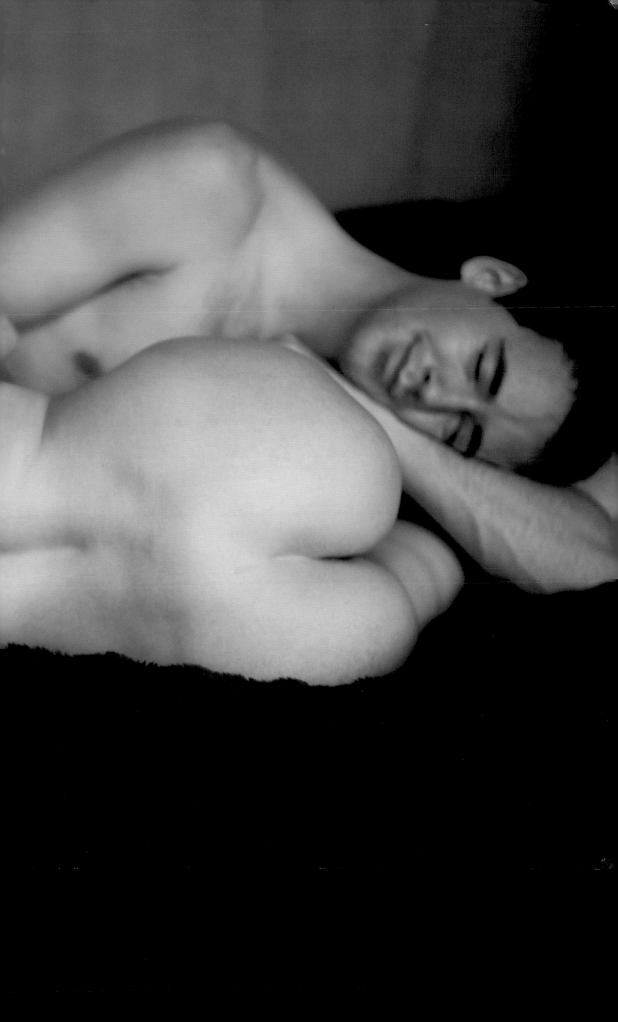

on gourmet lovemaking

All of us, barring any physical limitations, are able to dance and sing — after a fashion. This, if you think about it, summarizes the justification for learning to make love. Love, in the same way as singing, is something to be taken spontaneously. On the other hand, the difference between Pavlova and the Palais de Danse, or opera and barbershop singing, is much less than the difference between sex as our recent ancestors came to accept it and sex as it can be.

At least we recognize this now (so that instead of worrying if sex is sinful, most people now worry whether they are "getting satisfaction" — one can worry about anything, given the determination). And there are now enough books about the basics; we are largely past the point of people worrying about the normality, possibility, and variety of sexual experience. This book is slightly different, in that there are now enough people who have those basics and want more depth of understanding, solid ideas, and inspiration.

To draw a parallel, chef-grade cooking doesn't happen naturally: it starts at the point where people know how to prepare and enjoy food, are curious about it and willing to take trouble preparing it, read recipe hints, and find they are helped by one or two techniques. It's hard to make mayonnaise by trial and error, for instance. Gourmet sex, as we define it, is the same — the extra one can get from comparing notes, using some imagination, trying way-out or new experiences, when one already is making satisfying love and wants to go on from there.

This book will likely attract four sorts of readers. First, there are those who don't fancy it, find it disturbing, and would rather stay the way they are — these should put it down, accept our apologies, and stay the way they are. Second, there are those who are with the idea, but don't like our choice of techniques — remember, it's a menu, not a rulebook.

Third, most people will use our notes as a personal one-couple notebook from which they might get ideas. In this respect we have tried to stay wide open. One of the original aims of this book was to cure the notion, born of non-discussion, that common sex needs are odd or weird; the whole joy of sex-with-love is that there are no rules, so long as you enjoy, and the choice is practically

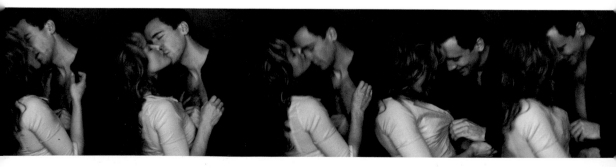

unlimited. We have, however, left out long discussion of very specialized sexual preferences; people who like these know already what they want to try.

The final group of readers are the hardy experimentalists, bent on trying absolutely everything. They too will do best to read this exactly like a cookbook – except that sex is safer in this respect, between lovers, in that you can't get obese or atherosclerotic on it, or give yourself ulcers. The worst you can get, given sensible safety precautions, is sore, anxious, or disappointed. However, one needs a steady basic diet of quiet, loving, night-and-morning intercourse to stand this experimentation on, simply because, contrary to popular ideas, the more regular sex a couple has, the higher the deliberately contrived peaks – just as the more you cook routinely, the better and the more reliable banquets you can stage.

One specific group of readers deserves special note. If you are disabled in any way, don't stop reading. A physical disability is not an obstacle to fulfilling sex. In counseling disabled people, one repeatedly finds that the real disability isn't a mechanical problem but a mistaken idea that there is only one "right" – or enjoyable – way to have sex. The best approach is probably to go through the book with your partner, marking off the things you can do. Then pick something appealing that you think you can't quite do, and see if there is a strategy you can develop together. Talking to other couples where one partner has a problem similar to yours is another resource.

In sum, the people we are addressing are the adventurous and uninhibited lovers who want to find the limits of their ability to enjoy sex. That means we take some things for granted – having intercourse naked and spending time over it; being able and willing to make it last, up to a whole afternoon on occasion; having privacy; not being scared of things like genital kisses; not being obsessed with one sexual trick to the exclusion of all others; and, of course, loving each other.

As the title implies, this book is about love as well as sex: you don't get high-quality sex on any other basis – either you love each other before you come to want it, or, if you happen to get it, you love each other because of it, or both. Just as you can't cook without heat, you can't make love without feedback. By feedback, we mean the right mixture of stop and go, tough and tender, exertion and affection. This comes by empathy and long mutual knowledge. Anyone

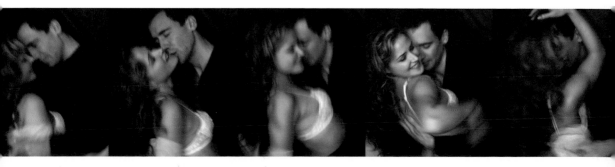

who expects to get this in a first attempt with a stranger is an optimist, or a neu-rotic — if they do, it's what used to be called love at first sight, and isn't expend-able: "skill," or variety, is no substitute. Also, one can't teach tenderness.

The starting point of all lovemaking is close bodily contact; love has been defined as the harmony of two souls, and the contact of two epiderms. At the same time, we might as well plan our menu so that we learn to use the rest of our equipment. That includes our feelings of identity, forcefulness, and so on, and all of our fantasy needs. Luckily, sex behavior in humans is enormously elastic (it has had to be, or we wouldn't be here), and also nicely geared to help us express most of the needs that society or our upbringing have corked up.

Elaboration in sex is something we need rather specially and it has the advantage that if we really make it work, it makes us more, not less, receptive to each other as people. This is the answer to anyone who thinks that con-scious effort to increase our sex range is "mechanical" or a substitute for real human relationship — we may start that way, but it's an excellent entry to learning that we are people and relating to each other as such. There may be other places we can learn to express all of ourselves, and do it mutually, but there aren't many.

Those are the assumptions on which this book is based. Granted this, there are two modes of sex — the duet and the solo — and a good concert alternates between the two. The duet is a cooperative effort aiming at simultaneous orgasm, or at least one orgasm each, and complete, untechnically planned release. This, in fact, needs skill, and can be built up from more calculated "love-play" until doing the right thing for both of you becomes fully automatic. This is the basic sexual meal.

The solo, by contrast, is when one partner is the player and the other the instrument. The aim of the player is to produce results on the other's pleasure experience as extensive, unexpected, and generally wild as his or her skill allows — to blow them out of themselves. The player doesn't lose control, though he or she can get wildly excited by what is happening to the other. The instrument does lose control — in fact, with a responsive instrument and a skillful performer, this is the concerto situation — and if it ends in an uncontrollable ensemble, so much the better. All the elements of music and dance are involved — rhythm,

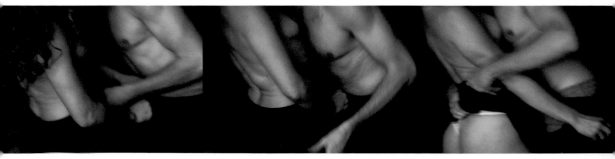

mounting tension, tantalization, even forcefulness: "I'm like the executioner," said the lady in the Persian poem, "but where he inflicts intolerable pain I will only make you die of pleasure." There is indeed an element of infliction in the solo mode, which is why some lovers dislike it and others overdo it, but no major lovemaking is complete without some solo passages.

The antique idea of the woman as passive and the man as performer used to ensure that he would show off playing solos on her, and early marriage manuals perpetuated this idea. Today, she is herself the soloist par excellence, whether in getting him excited to start with, or in controlling him and showing off all her skills. Solo recitals are not, of course, necessarily separate from intercourse. Apart from leading into it, there are many coital solos – for the woman astride, for example – while mutual masturbation or genital kisses can be fully fledged duets. Solo response can be electrifyingly extreme in the quietest people. Skilfully handled by someone who doesn't stop for yells of murder but does know when to stop, a woman can get orgasm after orgasm, and a man can be kept hanging just short of climax to the limit of human endurance. The solo-given orgasm, whether from her or from him, is unique – neither bigger nor smaller in either sex than a full duet but different; sharper but not so round. And most people who have experienced both like to alternate them. Trying to say how they differ is a little like describing wine. Differ they do, however, and much depends on cultivating and alternating them.

Top-level enjoyment doesn't have to be varied, it just often is. In fact, being stuck rigidly with one sex technique usually means anxiety. In this book we have not, for example, focused on coital postures to the exclusion of all else. The common positions are now familiar to most people from writing and pictures if not from trial – the more extreme ones, as a rule, should be spontaneous, but few of them have marked advantages. This explains the apparent emphasis in this book on extras – the "sauces and pickles." That said, individuals who, through a knot in their psyche, are obliged to live on sauce and pickle only are unfortunate in missing the most sustaining part of the meal – exclusive obsessions in sex are very like living exclusively on horseradish sauce through allergy to beef; fear of horseradish sauce, however, as indigestible, unnecessary, and immature is another hang-up, namely puritanism.

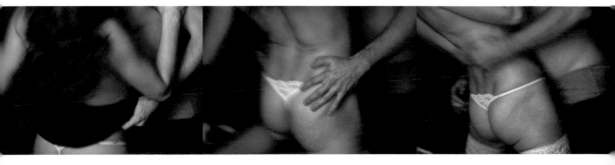

One of the things still missing from the essence of sexual freedom is the unashamed ability to use sex as play. In the past, ideas of maturity were nearly as much to blame as old-style moralisms about what is normal or perverse. We are all immature, and have anxieties and aggressions. Coital play, like dreaming, may be a programmed way of dealing acceptably with these, just as children express their fears and aggressions in games. Adults are unfortunately afraid of playing games, dressing up, and acting scenes. It makes them self-conscious: something horrid might get out. In this regard, bed is the place to play all the games you have ever wanted to play — if adults could become less self-conscious about such "immature" needs, we should have fewer deeply anxious people. If we were able to transmit the sense of play that is essential to a full, enterprising, and healthily immature view of sex between committed people, we would be performing a mitzvah: playfulness is a part of love that could be a major contribution to human happiness.

But still the main dish is loving, un-self-conscious sexual pleasure of all kinds — long, frequent, varied, ending with both parties satisfied, but not so full they can't face another light course, and another meal in a few hours. The pièce de résistance is good old face-to-face matrimonial, the finishing-off position, with mutual orgasm, and starting with a full day or night of ordinary tenderness. Other ways of making love are special in various ways, and the changes of timbre are infinitely varied — complicated ones are for special occasions, or special uses like holding off an over-quick male orgasm, or are things that, like pepper steak, are stunning once a year but not staples.

There are, after all, only two "rules" in good sex, apart from the obvious one of not doing things that are silly, antisocial, or dangerous. One is: "Don't do anything you don't really enjoy," and the other is: "Find out your partner's needs and don't balk at them if you can help it." In other words, a good giving and taking relationship depends on a compromise (so does going to a show — if you both want the same thing, fine; if not, take turns and don't let one partner always dictate). This can be easier than it sounds, because unless their partner wants something they find actively off-putting, real lovers get a reward not only from their own satisfaction but also from seeing the other respond and become satisfied. Most wives who don't like Chinese food will eat it occasionally for the pleasure of seeing a Sinophile husband enjoy it, and vice versa.

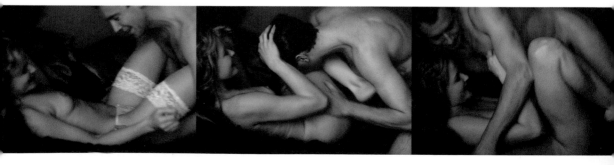

Partners who won't do this over specific sex needs are usually balking not because they have tried it and it's a turnoff (many experimental dishes are nicer than you expected), but through ignorance of the range of human needs, plus being scared if these include things like forcefulness, cultivating extragenital sensation, or role-playing, which previous social mythology pretended weren't there. Reading a full list of the unscheduled accessory sex behaviors that some normal people find helpful might be thought a necessary preliminary to any extended sexual relationship.

Couples should match up their needs and preferences (though people don't find these out at once); you won't get to some of our suggestions or understand them until you have learned to respond. It's a mistake to run so long as walking is such an enchanting and new experience, and you may be happy pedestrians who match automatically. Where a rethink really helps is at the point where you have gotten used to each other socially (sex needs aren't the only ones that need matching up between people who live together), and feel that the surface needs repolishing. If you think that sexual relations are over-rated, the surface does need repolishing, and you haven't paid enough attention to the wider use of your sexual equipment as a way of communicating totally. The traditional expedient at the point where the surface gets dull is to trade in the relationship and start all over in an equally uninstructed attempt with someone else, on the off chance of getting a better match-up by random choice. This is emotionally wasteful, and you usually repeat the same mistakes; better by far to repolish.

As to practicalities, we suggest couples either read the book together or (perhaps even better) read it separately, marking passages for the other partner's attention. This works wonders if – as is often the case – you don't really talk easily about sexual needs, or are afraid of sounding tactless.

Finally, if you don't like the repertoire or if it doesn't square with yours, never mind; the aim of *The Joy of Sex* is to stimulate your creative imagination. Sex books can only suggest techniques in order to encourage you to experiment. You can preface your own ideas with "this is how we play it," and play it your own way. But by that time, when you will have tried all your own creative sexual fantasies, you won't need books.

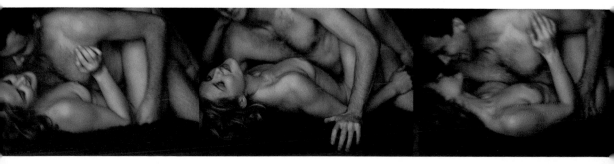

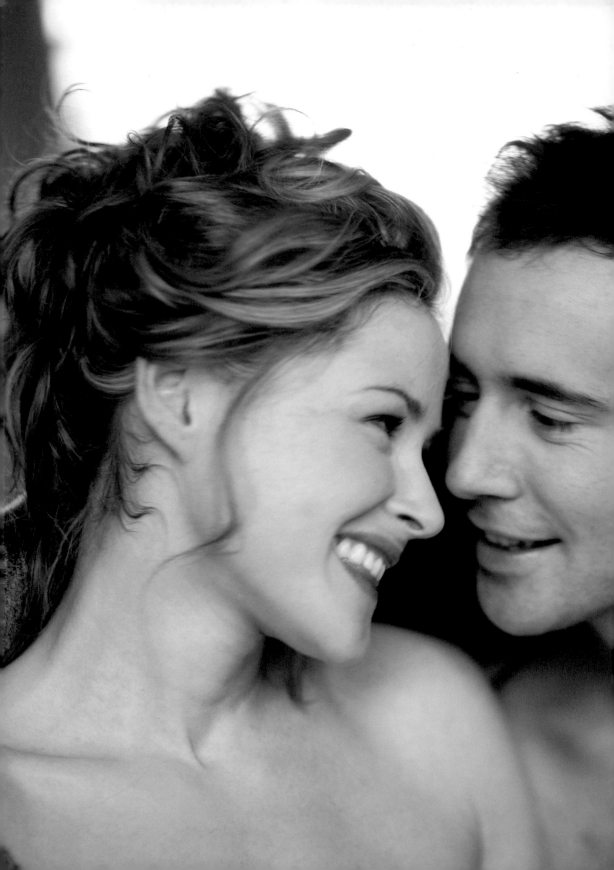

ingredients

tenderness

This, in fact, is what the whole book is about. It doesn't exclude extremely forceful games (though many people neither need nor want these), but it does exclude clumsiness, heavy-handedness, lack of feedback, spitefulness, and non-rapport generally. Tenderness is shown fully in the way you touch each other. What it implies at root is a constant awareness of what your partner is feeling, plus the knowledge of how to heighten that feeling, gently, toughly, slowly, or fast, and this can only come from an inner state of mind between the two of you. No really tender person can simply turn over and go to sleep afterwards.

Many if not most inexperienced men, and some women, are just naturally clumsy — either through haste, anxiety, or lack of sensing how the other sex feels — so don't grab breasts, stick fingers into the vagina, bend the penis, or (and this goes for both sexes) misplace bony parts of your anatomy. More women respond to very light than to very heavy stimulation — just brushing pubic or skin hairs will usually do far more than a whole-hand grab. At the same time, don't be frightened — neither of you is made of glass. Women, by contrast, often fail to use enough pressure, especially in hand work, though the light, light variety is a sensation on its own.

Start very gently, making full use of the skin surface, and work up. Stimulus toleration in any case increases with sexual excitement and even hard blows can become excitants (though not for everyone). This loss of pain sense disappears almost instantly with orgasm, so don't go on too long, and be extra gentle as soon as he or she has come.

If we could teach tenderness, most of this book would be superseded. If you are really heavy-handed, a little practice with inanimate surfaces, dress fastenings, and so on will help. Strength is a turn-on in sex, but it isn't expressed in clumsy hand work, bear hugs, and brute force — at least not as starters. If there is a problem here, remember you both can talk.

Few people want to be in bed on any terms with a person who isn't basically tender, and most people are delighted to be in bed with the right person who is. The ultimate test is whether you can bear to find the person there when you wake up. If you are actually pleased, then you can be sure that you are onto the right thing.

tenderness
a constant awareness of what your partner is
feeling, plus the knowledge of how to heighten
that feeling, gently, toughly, slowly, or fast

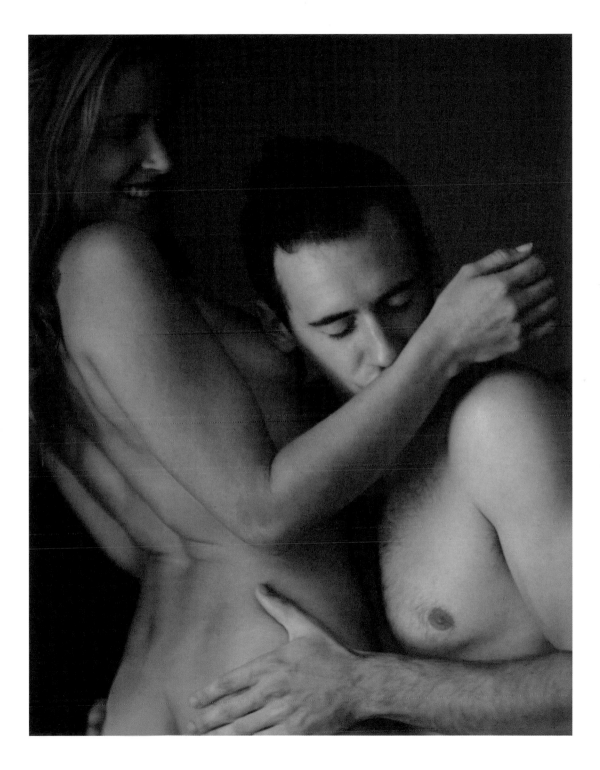

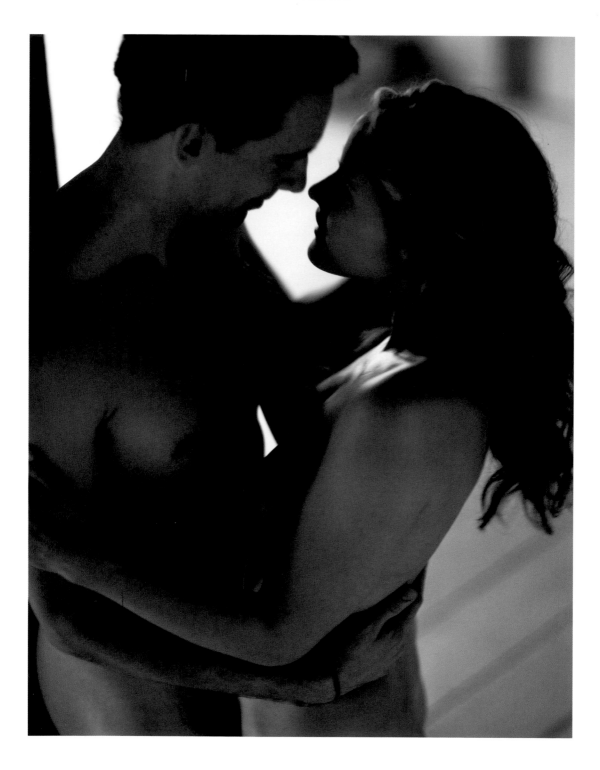

nakedness

The normal state for lovers who take their work at all seriously, at least as a basic requisite. They don't so much start clothed, and shed what they must, as start naked, and add any extras they need.

Nakedness doesn't mean lack of ornament. A woman may take off all her clothes, but put on all her jewels – the only practical need, as with wristwatches, is to see they don't catch or scratch. This is for daylight; it is difficult to sleep in them. For night, an increase in the value put on love-making is probably the main reason that many people now sleep naked. The only exception may be after; warm bodies tend to stick, and a blotter worn by one or other can add to comfort.

Nudists used to be associated with health fanatics enjoying a strict regime of cold showers and vigorous sports. Now, thank goodness, a more relaxed attitude prevails. Today, nudity is natural, not a ritual.

Organized "nudism" in most countries is a family affair. This is probably a good idea; the nudity of one's own parents can be worrying to some children, and shouldn't be overdone. There is, however, a lot to be said for the opportunity to look at men and women in general under unforced conditions; it is the discharge of residual anxiety of this sort about our body acceptability that probably makes group nudity so relaxing, rather than the opportunity to get an all-over tan. There is also evidence that children brought up in a naturist environment may be more responsible when faced with sexual opportunities and asked to make sexual choices. You should be able to pick a naturist club to taste – they offer facilities for open-air naked-ness, which are hard to organize at home, and are universally tough on sexual advances, which makes for an almost uniquely relaxed atmosphere.

nakedness
the normal state for lovers who
take their work at all seriously

women (by her for him)

Women, like men, have direct physical responses, sure – science proves that we get turned on just as much as you and as quickly; it's simply that traditionally we have been discouraged. But our triggers are different (breasts and skin first, please, not a direct grab at the clitoris), and can't be short-circuited. It matters to us who is doing what, far more than it does to most men. The fact that, unlike you, we can't be visibly turned off and lose erection often confuses men into hurrying things or missing major resources.

It isn't true that nudity, erotica, and so on don't excite us – probably the difference is that they aren't overriding things and that we don't separate them from emotions as easily as you do. Is it fair, I wonder, to give a simple instance? You, sir, can make orgiastically satisfactory love with a near stranger in half an hour flat. But please don't think for that reason that you can do the same for a woman who loves you personally if, at the end of the half-hour, you turn over and go straight to sleep. Granted this, however, there are common reactions.

Granted this difference, however, there are common reactions. We seem to be less heavily programmed than you for specific turn-ons, but once we see one of these working on a man we care about, we soon program it into our own response, and can be less rigid and more experimental because of this ability.

Often, if we seem underactive, it's because we are wary of doing the wrong thing with that particular man, like touching up his penis when, in fact, he is trying not to ejaculate – tell us if you see us at a loss. The penis isn't a "weapon" for us so much as a shared possession – it's less the size than its personality, unpredictable movements, and moods that make up the turn-on. We like penetration because it makes us feel close to you – but don't feel put down if we don't then necessarily climax through it alone (*see* her orgasm, pages 190–1); work with that rather than being discouraged by it.

Another important thing is the tough-tender mixture: obviously strength is a turn-on, but clumsiness (elbows in eyes, twisted fingers, for instance) is the dead opposite. You never get anywhere by clumsy brutality; however brutal good lovemaking sometimes looks, the turn-on is strength-skill-control, not large bruises, and the ability to be tender with it. Some people ask "tough or tender?" but the mood shifts so fast that you have got to be able to sense it. Surely it's possible – because some lovers do it – to read this balance from the feel of the woman.

No obsessive views about reciprocity – who comes on top and so on evens out during the passing of time: there can be long spells when we are happy to let you do the work, and others when we need to control everything ourselves and get an extra kick from seeing how we make you respond.

Women aren't "submissive" any more than men – if we have knuckled under in the past, it's only through social pressures. If we are dominant, we don't always act it out in bed by wearing spurs and cracking a whip. Men have a real advantage here in the constructive use of play (and can help women to act it out too). Since we all have some aggressions, good sex can be wildly forceful, but still never cruel.

As for sexual equality, nobody can possibly be a good lover without regarding their partner as a person and an equal. That is really all there is to be said on the matter.

Our sense of smell is the keener – don't oversaturate early on with masculine odors; just before orgasm is probably the time for full odor contact. Our own smell excites us as well as yours.

We learn, over a period of time, that the sort of hand- and mouth work that men like varies enormously. Some like it very rough, some hate it anything but extremely gentle, others in between. There is no way for us to tell except by asking and being told – therefore it's up to you to say what you like or you may get the opposite; remember that we love to know how to be good for you.

Some men are extraordinarily passive, or unimaginative, or inhibited, and – oddly – when they are any of these things, we don't become correspondingly forceful. We may long to do things and feel thoroughly frustrated, but we won't show it in most cases. So a woman's lovemaking will only be as good as her partner's and, more important, she will resent any man who is unexciting, not only because he is unexciting, but also because she will know she has been unexciting too.

Finally, you should never presume that what excites one woman sexually will work just as well on another woman. Women probably do differ sexually rather more than men, because of the greater complexity of our sexual apparatus (breasts, skin, and so on as well as pussy). Never assume that you don't need to relearn for each person. This is also true for a woman with a new man, but perhaps a little less so.

men (by him for her)

We often wish that women's sexuality was like ours, even though we know it isn't. Our sexual response is far brisker and more automatic: it's triggered easily by things, like putting a coin in a vending machine. Consequently, women and parts of women provide automatic sexual stimulus for us; your clothes, breasts, odor, and so on aren't what we love instead of you   simply

men (by him for her)
the most valued thing in
lovemaking is "the divine
gift of lechery"

the things we need in order to set sex in motion and express love. You seem to find this hard to understand.

Secondly, most though not all male feeling is ultimately centered in the last inch of the penis (though you can, if you start intelligently, teach us female-type sensitivity all over the surface of our skin). And unlike yours, our sexuality depends on a positive performance – we have to be turned on to achieve an erection, and not turned off, in order to function; we can't be passively "taken." This matters intensely to men at both a biological and a personal level; sexual success is what makes us feel worthwhile. It explains why we are emphatically penis-centered and tend to open the proceedings with genital play, probably before you are ready and when you would much rather wait to get in the mood. Genital approach is how we get into the mood.

You need to understand these reactions, as we need to understand yours. A woman's concern about being a sex object misses the point – sure, the woman and the various parts of her are sex objects, but most men ideally would wish to be treated piecemeal in the same way. Thus, the most valued thing, from you, in actual lovemaking, is intuition of these object reactions, and direct initiative – starting the play, taking hold of the penis, giving genital kisses ahead of being asked; being an initiator, a user of your stimu-

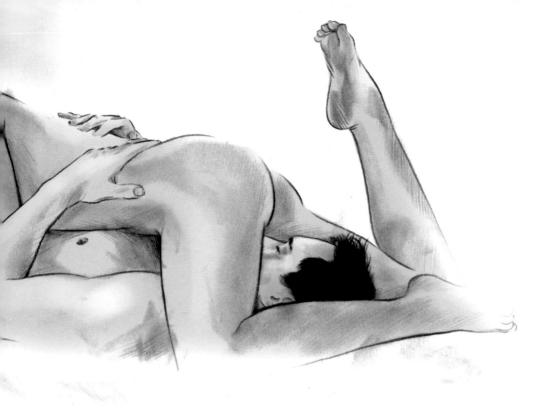

latory equipment. This is hard to put in simple terms; it is what is meant by "the divine gift of lechery" – the art of sensing turn-ons and going along with them for the partner's response. It isn't the same for the two sexes because male turn-ons are concrete, while many female turn-ons are situational and atmospheric. Remember too that we may simply be tired of having to deliver, in life as well as in bed, and your taking over doesn't just offer us the ultimate compliment, it also gives us the opportunity to relax and enjoy. Sex may be about the only place in our lives where we get to be held and nurtured.

Personal folklore apart, what the male turn-on equipment requires is the exact reverse of a virgin or a passively recipient instrument – not a demand situation, because that in itself can threaten a turnoff due to feelings of inadequacy, but a skill situation; I can turn you on, and turn myself on in doing so, and from that point we play it both ways and together. You can't, of course, control your turn-ons any more than we can, but it helps if you have some male-type object reactions, like being excited by the sight of a penis, or hairy skin, or by the man stripping, or by physical kinds of play (just as it helps if we have some sense of atmosphere). It's the active woman who understands our reactions, plays on them, and leads them out while keeping her own who is the ideal lover.

hormones

The fuel in the sex machine, keeping desire, arousal, and performance ticking over, as well as driving affection and love. For the most part, they form a constant underpinning of mood, supporting though never replacing the honest-to-goodness sexual diesel generated by enthusiastic lovers.

A peak or a valley, on the other hand, can impact. Sexually, the crucial fuel is testosterone, for her as well as for him. His will peak during his twenties, then settle into a more or less consistent pattern, dipping over the course of a long-term relationship and rising in a new one; no excuse for straying, but a possible explanation of the temptation to do so. With age, it will gently decline — but rarely enough to cause problems; if his erection is failing, that's reason for action, not resignation.

In her, testosterone has the same effect, raising desire, demand, and energy; in the last third of her menstrual month, when levels of the hormone are high, try more urgent, fighting sex. Around the menopause, as estrogen drops away and testosterone levels stay high, she may find to her delight a lust that lasts for months or years — a second adolescence of which she can take full advantage.

Oxytocin, the "cuddle hormone," both bonds partners in affection and makes them less likely to want to be sexual — one reason why the post-orgasmic default is to hug rather than go for a second bout. Add in prolactin, the "done that, time to rest" hormone also released at orgasm, to explain why, for him in particular, the default may well be to sleep. Prolactin is released when breast-feeding too, another reason why post-partum she may be utterly turned off all things sexual — just as the contraceptive pill, breast-feeding, and stress may imbalance her general hormone levels, with the same low-desire result. But never be held hostage — hormones may affect mood, but they can't overrule action; clear thinking, reassuring communication, and making love regardless are often enough to offset imbalances.

These notes are mainly included here for interest and understanding — all genuine lovers will want to know what's under the hood in order to make the car purr more sweetly — but largely there are no bedroom applications. If the machine falters, however, science is increasingly able to supply an answer; see your doctor.

preferences

More of us than we may think have a wide sexual range – that is to say, are able to respond sexually to either gender. Yes, many recognize who they are early in life and never shift. But adolescents often experiment before settling, and adults dream; same-sex relationships are in the top three sexual fantasies for heterosexuals, and some of the most surprising people – like Hans Christian Andersen – live out such dreams in real life. Preferences are not a choice that can be overridden in the long term; you may like both sexes, but if you don't, the irrelevant one simply doesn't smell right and there is no negotiating that.

If you occasionally wonder – as opposed to having strong and clear desires in a particular direction – you are probably not gay but curious. If you have strong, clear desires, don't agonize but talk it through; ringing a gay or lesbian help line won't mean you are persuaded or presupposed into it, but will mean you speak to someone who has asked themselves the same questions as you have and found appropriate answers. Your own answer, once found, could transform your sex life and also your life in general; passion can flow and activities that seemed off-putting with one gender can, with the other, feel natural and fulfilling. Surely it doesn't need saying that the joy of sex is rooted in knowing who you really are.

As to the whole political agenda, happily in most countries all of the above is not the "problem" it was when this book was first written, though in most cultures it's still a challenge and in others it's still actively against the law, either secular or religious. We, however, believe that one person's flavor of sexuality is no one else's business; everyone should be free to follow their inclinations without fear or favor. If you don't, you not only waste your own life pretending to be someone you aren't, you also potentially waste the life of a partner who knows there is something not quite right but can't pinpoint it. Whatever your preferences, be honest with yourself and your beloved, and never think you can "cure" a partner of their own preference by imposing yours upon them.

This book is written for the straight reader but, within the context of a loving relationship, behaviors borrowed from the whole range of possible preferences can have their uses. Don't dismiss (or judge) anything until you have tried it at least once.

confidence

It is, surely, a self-fulfilling prophecy that the more confident you are, the more you will enjoy sex. This is not about arrogance – the assumption that one is God's gift will be an instant turnoff, particularly to women, if only because they know with that sort of mental map a man won't have bothered to learn enough to be even moderately useful. At the other end of the extreme, a partner who starts off lacking in confidence only proves delightful if they ultimately benefit from care and feeding; lasting and insistent insecurity is draining in bed and out of it.

But true sexual confidence – being relaxed, knowledgeable about oneself, willing to learn about another, ready to ask for what's needed, happy to take charge, and unwobbled by either failure or rejection – makes for that ultimate in sexual partners, one who is able both to give and receive with an equal abundance of pleasure.

This has nothing to do with looks. Nowadays, almost all women – and an increasing number of men – are scared of being spurned on that count, but this is because the media manipulates body image. If you don't love your body, change your mind; if your partner doesn't love your body, change your partner. Note to her: men are almost always more focused on sensation and the feelings of acceptance that sex gives than on your size, shape, or degree of firmness. If he has ever hugged you clothed, he already knows your shape; if when you are unclothed he has an erection, then he not only accepts but lusts after it. Note to him: women care hardly at all about shape, so relax please.

He, however, may have other insecurities. He is asked to demonstrate potency in much more obvious ways than she is, and the men's magazines may have convinced him that unless he can do so he will be rejected. But in terms of pure erection, there are always other ways – and for most women those ways are just as acceptable, certainly on an occasional basis. If generally nervous, the answer is to end up in bed only with a partner one is relaxed with and then try things out. As with all human activities, the way to mastery is through play.

Whatever one's size, experience, and ability – or disability – good sex is one of the most powerful confidence-builders because it places each partner right in the center of the other's attention; beyond that, genuine compliments, demonstrated affection, and a total lack of comparison will complete the magic spell. She says: "Show me that you think I'm beautiful and everything else follows." His words may be different, but the essential message will be the same.

cassolette

French for perfume box. The natural perfume of a clean woman: her great-est sexual asset after her beauty (some would say greater than that). It comes from the whole of her – hair, skin, breasts, armpits, genitals, and the clothing she has worn: it is her own signature scent and no two women are the same in this respect. Men have a natural perfume too, which women are aware of, but while a man can be infatuated with a woman's personal perfume, women on the whole simply tend to notice if a man smells right or wrong. Wrong means not so much unpleasant as intangibly not for them. Often their awareness of a man includes conditioned extras such as work odors or aftershave.

Because it's so important, she needs to guard her own personal perfume carefully and learn to use it as part of her powers of attraction as skillfully as she uses the rest of her body. (We now know the science behind all this – pheromones, a kind of biological speed-bonding, making one attractive, relaxing a potential partner, creating mood. They say,"I'm interested . . . I'm interesting.") In particular, a woman's personal perfume can be a long-range weapon (nothing seduces a man more reliably, and this can happen subliminally), but at the same time a skillful man can read it, if he is an olfactory type, and if he knows her, to determine when she is sexually excited.

Susceptibility and consciousness of human clean perfumes vary in both sexes. Women have the keener sense of smell, but men respond to it more as an attractant. Whether these are inborn differences, like inability to smell asparagus, or whether they are due to unconscious blocking-out, we don't know. Some children can't understand the point of blind man's buff because they know by smell who is touching them: some women can smell that they are pregnant. Men can't smell some chemicals related to musk unless they have a shot of female sex hormone. Far more human loves and antipathies are based on smell than our deodorant-and-aftershave culture admits. Many people, especially women, say that when it's a question of bed or not-bed, they let their noses lead them.

Which means it's sad that, culturally, we are conditioned to deodorize and perfume. Better by far would be soap and water, although the unfortu-nates who sweat profusely may well have problems. A mouthful of aluminium chloride in an armpit is one of the biggest disappointments bed can afford, and a truly deodorized partner would be another. If smell (and taste) do become unpleasant, it's probably a shift of diet or an infection; both can be cleared up, and should be done so in short order. There is no excuse for bad breath or the unilateral eating of garlic. Where lovemaking regularly happens at the end of a long, hot, or hard day, create a ritual of showering together beforehand. If you find each other's perfume becoming distasteful long term, however, it may be a reflection of a more emotional distaste. Take it seriously.

Many women shave their armpit hair, conditioned as they are by the idea that hairlessness is sexy. Opinions are divided on this one – fashion dictates armpits should be bare, but hairs catch our pheromonal scent. This could be played as an argument for more body hair in general, but men's facial hair doesn't have the day-to-day importance of a woman's little tufts. These are antennae and powder puffs to introduce herself in a room, or in love-making. They are there to brush the man's lips with; he can do the same more circumspectly. Kissing deeply in the armpit leaves a partner's perfume with you.

In the genital kiss, start with the lips covered, then brush the closed lips, then open her; when she gives the kiss to a man, she proceeds in the same order. It's the fullest way to become aware of each other, even before you start to touch. She will feel much more at ease with this if he says clearly that he likes her scent and taste. Many women labor under the belief that their natural odor, particularly the pussy scent, is too strong. He can reverse this more or less instantly by showing enthusiasm.

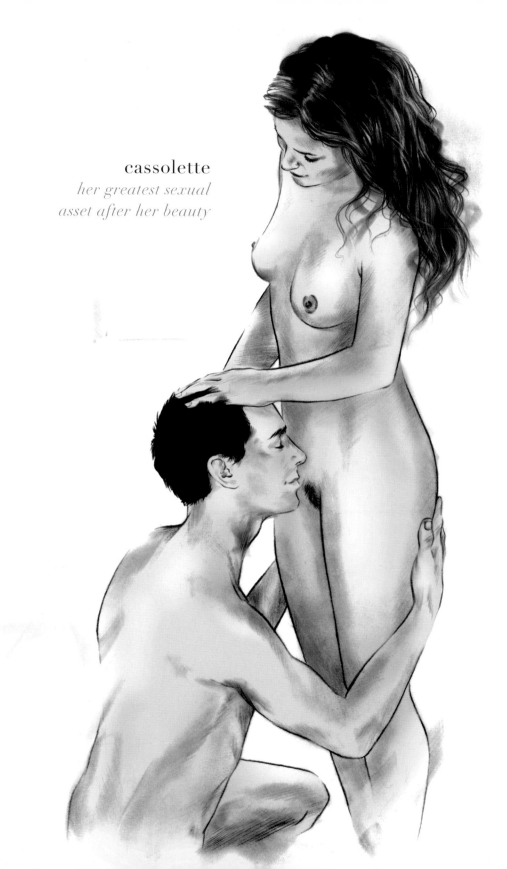

cassolette
*her greatest sexual
asset after her beauty*

vulva

Her external parts, the equivalent of scrotum and penile skin for him, and beautifully immortalized in feminist artist Judy Chicago's exhibition *The Dinner Party*; thirty-nine vulval images symbolizing thirty-nine inspirational women. Can be stroked, sucked, squeezed, licked, softly stimulated with a vibrator — go up one side and down the other. Her perineum — between vagina and anus — is as sensitive as his; tease gently with a fingertip. The U-spot (*see* trigger points, page 153), between clitoris and vagina, can also be gently pressed in circular movements — use a careful knuckle or the tip of his penis; an unerect penis will give different sensations from an erect one. If she is sensitive post-climax, this will help her scale the peak again.

vulva
can be stroked, sucked,
squeezed, licked, softly
stimulated with a vibrator

She may be insecure about the way she looks here — color, thickness, and size — but this is just one more reflection of the fact that most genital images we see have been doctored. New or growing lumps or bumps, however, like rashes or pain, need attention. The current fashion for "tidying" labia surgically is a mutilation; in cultures less primitive than ours, women do the opposite, actively stretching their labia, then proudly folding them into origami shapes.

vagina

As magic as the penis, and to some males slightly scary: luckily, few anxieties survive closer acquaintance, but they are involved in certain male hang-ups. Prudes treat it as if it was radioactive – "All magic," said a Papuan wizard, "radiates from it as fingers do from a hand" – and a lot of put-downs of women throughout history grew from this kind of Freudian undergrowth.

This is sad, for the vagina to her is as powerful yet vulnerable as the penis is to him, the source of reassuring menstrual blood, thudding orgasms, longed-for birth. Theoretically, only the first third of the vagina is truly sensitive; as a symbol of her openness and femininity, however, the whole of it is at the heart of her sexuality.

Normally slightly moist, or women would squeak when they walk, the vagina wets more or less copiously with sexual excitement; some women also ejaculate at orgasm, though that's certainly not universal (see trigger points, page 153). Apart from this, any staining, discharge, rash, bleeding, or pain indicates infection and needs checking out; have regular Pap smears and a vaccination too, please, to protect against cervical cancer. The normal vaginal odor varies greatly between women and between times, but should always be pleasant and sexually exciting. For care and maintenance, don't douche – it destroys not only healthy secretions but also the pheromones that attract him. A healthy vagina self-cleans.

Whether or not he has ever explored a woman's pussy in detail, with fingers, eyes, and tongue, he should make sure he explores hers. She should learn to kiss with it – she has two mouths to his one.

clitoris

The first edition of this book commented that "the phallic-minded male is inclined to make a reassuring rush for the clitoris." We now know that such a male would be absolutely correct; the clitoris and the phallus are in fact gender-adapted equals. Australian urologist Helen O'Connell's research shows that the average clitoris – both what's above the surface and the much bigger section buried in the pelvis – is quite as big as a flaccid penis, is made of exactly the same erectile tissue, has a penis-like shaft, and displays a tiny glans with its own foreskin. Smugly, it also has twice the number of nerve endings as its male counterpart.

Whether because of too little knowledge or too much distrust, society has never given the clitoris the same weight of symbolism as the penis. Those more aware, however, know that its role is to set light to the vagina as "pine shavings can be kindled to set a log of... wood on fire" (Freud).

Comedienne Carol Leifer put it more succinctly: "Making love to a woman is like buying real estate: location, location, location" (*see* clitoral pleasure, page 142). It is regrettable that some cultures feel the need to excise it — though Western cultures too, until very recently, used circumcision as a cure for "female problems."

As to its role in climax, there is surely no point in joining the "pro" or "con" debate; everyone has the right to experience an orgasm in as many ways as they want to and are able to. But it should be added that while many women don't ever orgasm easily through intercourse, few fail to orgasm through stimulation of the clitoris. It is, of course, the only human organ designed purely for pleasure.

mons pubis

The decorative fat pad situated over the female pubic bone that acts as a buffer in face-to-face intercourse, and which, more importantly, incorporates a layer of nerve endings that serve to transmit sensation to the rest of the area when it moves or is moved.

Many men are not aware, if they are oversold on direct clitoris stimulation, that most women can be brought to orgasm simply by holding this gently in the cupped hand and kneading or shaking it, before, without, or as well as putting a finger in the vagina (*see* pubic hair, pages 72–4).

He can either grasp it (it exactly fits the palm) or rest the heel of his hand on it while using the fingers on the labia, or he can cup the whole area, mons and closed labia, in palm and fingers; he can then practice seeing how much sensation he can produce with her lying completely closed. In return, she can grasp his mons, circling his penis with her fingers, her other hand on his scrotum — though typically the effect is not the same, some men find that it simply tickles.

breasts

"In our maturer years," wrote Erasmus Darwin, "when an object of vision is presented to us which bears any similitude to the form of the female bosom . . . we feel a general glow of delight, which seems to influence all our senses, and if the object be not too large we experience an attraction to embrace it with our lips as we did in early infancy the bosom of our mothers."

Breasts are the natural second target, but often the first one we reach. Just how sensitive they are, in men as well as in women, varies enormously, and according to physical state and mood. As with other sexual organs, size is unimportant in relation to sensitivity; if it still creates insecurity, however, fascinated attention is a more effective cure than surgery. Some breasts don't answer at all, even in the emphatically non-frigid; some answer to extremely gentle touches, some to very rough handling (but they are sensitive structures – don't let a need for forceful contact get the better of sound common sense).

Going round and round the nipple with the tongue tip or the glans, soft kneading with both hands, gentle biting, and sucking gently like a baby are the best gambits – she can do the same for him. (While there, both can occasionally check for suspicious lumps.)

If her breasts are big enough to meet, one can get a surprising degree of mutuality from intermammary intercourse. This is a good expedient on occasions when she doesn't feel like vaginal intercourse. She lies half flat on pillows, he kneels astride (big toe to her clitoris if she needs helping) with his foreskin, if he has one, fully retracted. Either he or she can hold the breasts together – wrap them around the shaft rather than rub the glans with them. It should protrude clear, just below her chin. Intercourse between the breasts is equally good in other positions – head to tail, or with her on top (especially if she has small breasts), or man sitting, woman kneeling; experiment accordingly. An orgasm from this position, if she gets one, is "round" like a full coital orgasm, and she feels it inside. Breast orgasms from licking and handling are "in between" in feel. His ejaculation this way gives her what's known as a "pearl necklace"; he should rub the semen well into her breasts when he has finished (*see* semen, page 62).

Breasts, vagina, and clitoris all at once make the fastest and most concentrated buildup of sensation once intercourse has begun, for some women at least. Many easily stimulated women can also experience a rather special pleasure from suckling a baby.

breasts
an orgasm from this
position is "round," and
she feels it inside

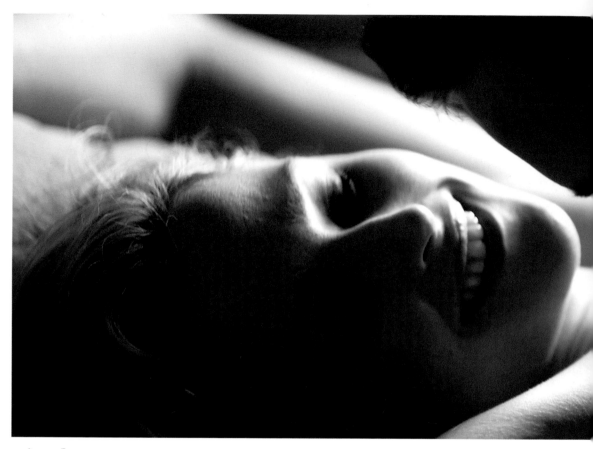

nipples

She says: "Unlike a man's nipples, a woman's can have a direct hotline to her clitoris and vagina. A man who can dial this correctly and will only take the time can do anything. Palm-brushing, eyelash-brushing, licking, and loud sucking like a baby can work wonders; the orgasms one gets from these are mind-blowing without detracting a jot from intercourse to come after. Please take time." He, meanwhile, can get a very special jolt from this, made more intense still if she is actually lactating; male suckling is more of a majority interest than you might think.

On him, rather than by him, stimulation is less likely to have an effect; few men can get a nipple orgasm, but try a stiff pair of feathers (*see* feathers, page 113) or very gentle fingertip friction – men's nipples easily get sore.

If the effect seems lacking, assiduous attention over time may help; try gentle circles with a toothbrush. There is no proof in the theory that caffeine creates temporary nipple sensitivity, but it's still worth a try. Fluctuating

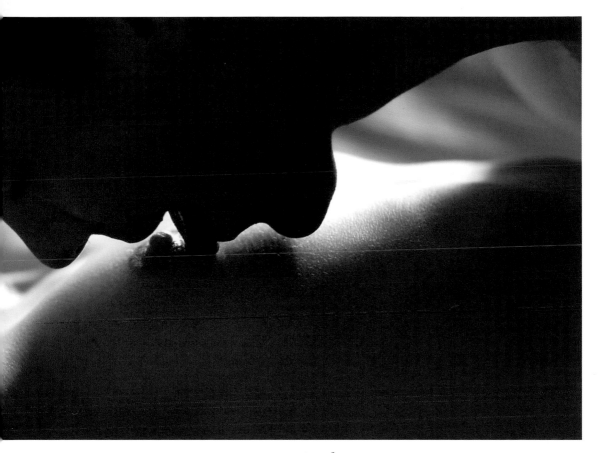

nipples
a direct hotline to her most sensitive parts

hormones before her period can turn sensitivity into discomfort, and if there is itching, swelling, bleeding, or discharge, get it checked out. This applies to him as well as to her.

If a partner likes pain, or to test the possibility without putting the question direct, pinch nipples lightly, then harder (never when sore, lactating, or newly pierced). The aim is a balance of pleasure and pain; after, once pressure is released, the whole body will be achingly sensitive for hours. If this appeals, move to nipple clamps (not clothes pegs, which aren't adjustable); a linked pair with one on each of his and her breasts also provides a neat accompaniment to any movements that create a gentle tug. When taken off, pinch with fingers, then release slowly to allow the blood to flow back in comfortably. Limit time on such play – 15 minutes is enough.

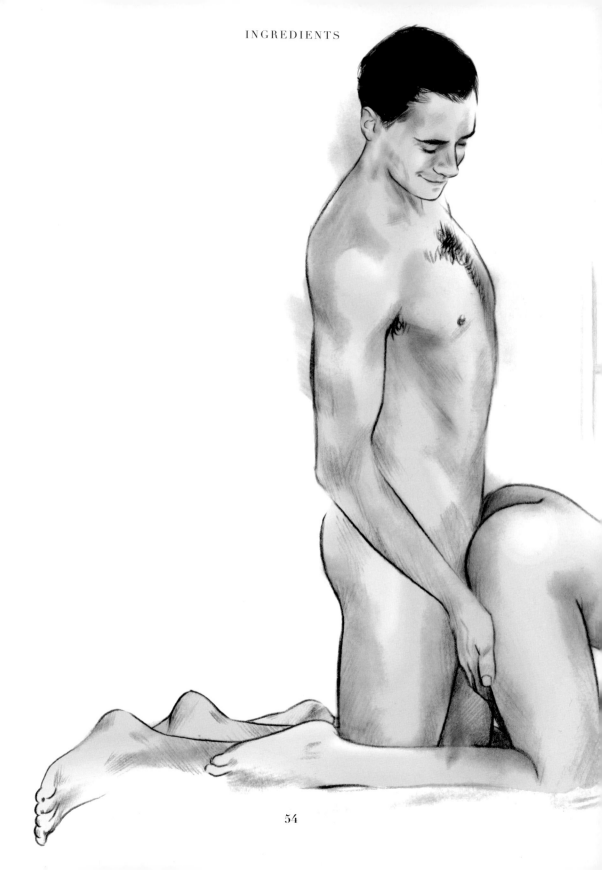

buttocks

Next in line after breasts, buttocks alternate with them as visual sex stimuli for different cultures and individuals. Actually the original primate focus, being brightly colored in most apes; apparently equally fancied by the Neanderthals, who produced some of the best Stone Age figurines.

The buttocks are a major erogenous zone in both sexes, though less sensitive than breasts because they have fewer nerves and a layer of fat, and so need stronger stimulation (holding, kneading, slapping, or even harder beating – *see* discipline, pages 265–7).

Intercourse from behind (*see* rear entry, pages 169–71) is a pleasure in itself, but be careful if she has a weak back. In any position the muscular movements of coitus stimulate the buttocks in both sexes, particularly if each holds the partner's rear fairly tightly, one cheek in each hand. These extra sensations are well worth cultivating deliberately. Visually, good buttocks are a turn-on in almost equal measure for both sexes.

buttocks
a turn-on in almost
equal measure for
both sexes

penis

Not only the essential piece of male equipment, even if it is often and expressively described as a "tool," the penis has more symbolic importance than any other human organ, as a dominance signal and, by reason of having a will of its own, generally a "personality." No point in reading all this symbolism back here, except to say that lovers will experience it, and find themselves treating the penis as something very like a third party. At one moment it's a weapon or a threat, at another something they share, like a child. Without going into psychoanalysis or biology, it's not a bad test of a love relationship if, while the penis is emphatically his, it also belongs to both of them. In any case, its texture, erectility, and so on are fascinating to both sexes, and its apparent autonomy, a little alarming.

Like the vagina, the penis collects anxieties and folklore, and is a focus for all sorts of magical manipulations. Male self-esteem and sense of identity tend to be located in it, as Samson's energy was in his hair. If it won't work, or worse, if she sends it up, or down, the results will be disastrous. This explains the irrational male preoccupation with penile size. Size has absolutely nothing to do with physical serviceability in intercourse, or – since female orgasm doesn't depend on getting deeply into the pelvis – with capacity to satisfy a partner, though many women are turned on by the idea of a large one, and a few say that they feel more (*see* size, pages 60–1). If anything, thickness matters more than length. Nor has flaccid size anything to do with erect size – a penis that is large when at rest simply enlarges less with erection. There is no way of artificially "enlarging" a penis.

Nor, except in very rare cases, is a penis too big for a woman – widthwise, the vagina will take a full-term baby. If his penis, whatever its length, knocks an ovary and hurts her, he shouldn't go in so far. A woman who says she is "too small" or "too tight" is usually making a statement about her arousal levels; she needs time, understanding, and foreplay. Shape also varies – the glans can be blunt or conical. This matters only in that the conical shape can make receptacle-tipped condoms uncomfortable through getting jammed in the tip.

Women who have really learned to enjoy sex are usually as fascinated by their lover's penis, size included, as men are by women's breasts, shape, odor, and feel, and learn to play with it fully and skillfully. Circumcised or not (*see* foreskin, page 61), it's a fascinating toy quite apart from its main use. There is a whole play scene connected with uncapping, stiffening, and handling it, making it pulsate or ejaculate, that is a major part of togetherness. This is equally important for the man – not only is it ego-boosting, but good hand- and mouth work practically guarantee a good sexual partner.

Care and maintenance: if he isn't circumcised, he will need to retract the foreskin fully for cleaning purposes, and if it won't retract beyond the corona all round the glans except at the front, get it seen to (correcting it involves a trifling operation with a blunt probe and doesn't necessarily mean that he needs circumcising). If it won't retract properly or is over-tight and gets stuck, get that attended to as well.

Slight asymmetry often develops with time – this does no harm unless it's pronounced or painful, in which case see a doctor. On the other hand, don't bend an erect penis or use a position in which it could get violently bent by accident. (This usually happens with the woman on top if she is careless near orgasm, or in putting him in, and he is just short of fully stiff – keep a little control here.) It is possible, though difficult, to fracture one of the two hydraulics contained in the shaft. This is very painful and can lead to pain or kinking on subsequent erection. The normal organ will stand up to extremely hard use, but not to these. (Avoid also silly tricks with suction and so on – *see* inflators, page 250.)

Sores, discharge, lumps, bumps, bleeding, and so on signal illnesses and need treatment. Even if you both have proof that you are free of all sexually transmitted diseases – if you aren't, condoms are mandatory – don't have oral intercourse with someone who has a herpes on the mouth; you can get recurrent herpes of the penis or the vulva, which is a nuisance.

If the foreskin is dry from masturbation or long retraction, saliva is the recommended lubricant. Commercial equivalents are now sold that make things more comfortable and add sensation, but steer clear of the ones that claim to slow down or speed up response; they can anesthetize or irritate him and, by association, her. If he has problems in this department, it's best to use less "quick-fix" methods (*see* hair-trigger trouble, page 185, and performance, pages 148–9).

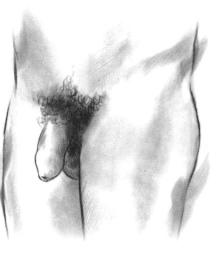

penis
has more symbolic importance
than any other human organ

penis
while the penis is
emphatically his, it also
belongs to both of them

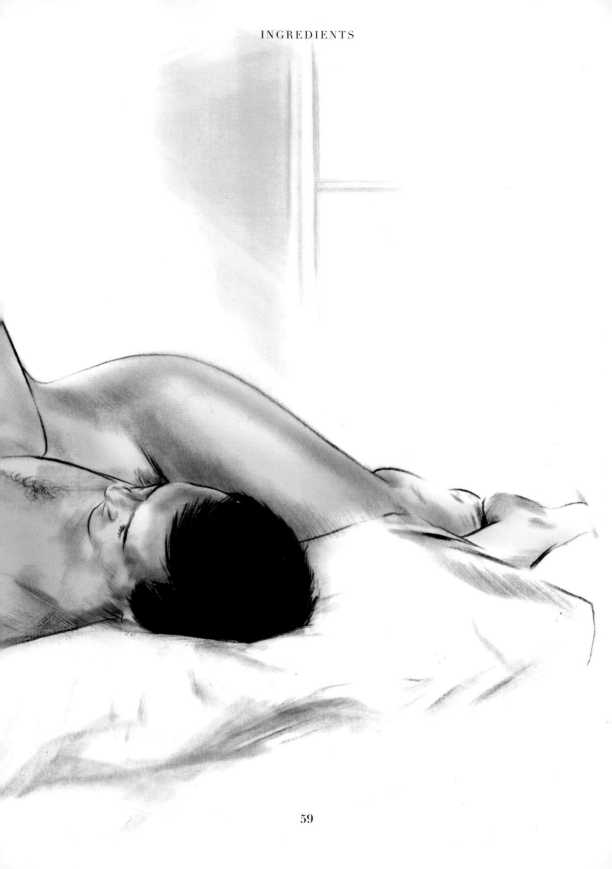

size

Preoccupation with the size of their genitals is about as common in men (it is a "dominance signal," like a deer's antlers) as sensitivity about their breasts and figure is in women. That, however, is its only importance in matters sexual. The "average" penis is just over five inches overall when erect and between three and four inches round, but penises come in all sizes – larger ones may be spectacular, but no more effective except as visual stimuli. Smaller ones work equally well in most positions – and may, as only the first few inches of the vagina are sensitive, actually work better than larger examples. In any case, she will almost always report that what matters is how it's used, not how big it is.

Non-erect size in the male is equally unimportant – some men before erection show no penile shaft at all, but extend to full size easily. The same applies to testicle weight – it varies, as does nose or mouth size, but has little to do with function. Small genitals are usually due to active muscles in the layer beneath the skin – a cold bath will shrink the best-endowed male down to Greek-statue proportions.

Accordingly, excessive preoccupation with size is an irrational anxiety, often created by the fact that men see their own penises as small because they are seen from above and other men's penises as large because they are seen from the front. Don't fall for the hype on lotions, potions, stretching exercises, or surgery – one can't reliably and safely increase size, any more than one can increase stature. She should learn not to comment on it except favorably; he should learn not to give it a second thought. The few cases where male genitalia are really infantile occur in conjunction with major gland disturbances and are treatable but rare.

All the above reassurance also applies to vaginal size. Few women are too small; lubricate, add lots of foreplay, wait until she has "ballooned" through arousal before penetrating. So long as she isn't hurting – in which case stop instantly – a tight woman gives the man extra-intense feelings. Nor is any vagina too large: if it seems a loose fit, switch to a posture in which her thighs are pressed together – from behind for best effect. Long term, do Kegel exercises (see *pompoir*, page 188) to keep muscles toned – though lots of sex works just as well and she will enjoy it more. Apart from postpartum stitching, surgery to tighten the vagina is usually a reflection of lack of confidence on her part or inappropriate demands on his.

Genital anatomy probably fixes which postures work best for a given couple, but no more than that. With rare exceptions, men and women are universally adapted. The only practical exception is in the case of a very big penis and a very small woman, in which case she should be careful on top, or she will knock an ovary (which feels very much like accidentally knocking a testicle does for a man), and he should avoid thrusting too hard until he knows he won't hurt her. As to the size of other structures, such as breasts, these may be individual turn-ons, but every build has its sexual opportunities built in: use them.

foreskin

Cutting off this structure is possibly the oldest human sexual ritual. It still persists – for cultural as well as supposed health reasons. Some believe that cancer of the penis and cervix is rarer when it's done (a myth) or that it slows down orgasm (for which there is no evidence). It probably doesn't make very much difference, either to masturbation or to intercourse – one normally retracts it anyway for all these purposes – though if he doesn't have one, there is a whole range of covered-glans nuances he can't recapture. Holding the skin back hard with the hand (her hand) during intercourse works for both the circumcised and uncircumcised as an accelerator, and offers a sensation of its own.

Women who have experienced both are divided – as they are over which looks sexier. Some find the circumcised glans "neater" and are even turned off by an unretracted prepuce as looking "feminine," while others love the sense of discovery that goes with retraction. If he is uncircumcised and she prefers the other, he can retract it – if vice versa, simply find other amusements. In terms of function, it's probably there for immunological protection and helpful for lubrication – the high density of nerve endings doesn't harm either.

While in the area, a word about the frenulum, the "little bridle" that connects the underside of the glans to the shaft. It is sensitive to stretching – it's probably this that creates the sensation during up-and-down hand work – and circumcision may tighten it or sometimes remove it altogether. If it's intact, try lubricated palm over glans, with thumb massaging frenulum and little finger directly on it circling smaller and smaller. Flick across with the tongue and apply sustained pressure while he simply relaxes. Reserve this technique, however, until he is ready to come more or less instantly.

In sum, the circumcised man isn't at any important disadvantage (or advantage), but many people prefer to be able to choose their egg with or without salt, and let their children do likewise.

scrotum

Basically, a sperm factory. The testes produce sperm; the scrotum is the control device to keep them producing it at the right temperature, moving up when he is cold and down when he is warm. No need to panic at asymmetry — it's normal for one testicle to be smaller and for the left one to hang slightly lower — though extraneous lumps or pain should be checked out immediately. It's also a highly sensitive skin area, and needs careful handling, since pressure on a testis is highly painful to its proprietor. Gentle tongue and finger work or cupping in the hand is about right, or try a fingertip along the visible center line and gentle teasing on the perineum between scrotum and anus. She can take it right into her mouth.

semen

There is no lovemaking without spilling this, on occasions at least. You can get it out of clothing or furnishings either with a stiff brush, when the stain has dried, or with a dedicated cleanser designed to remove blood. If you spill it over each other, massage it gently in. If you want a very copious ejaculate, he can masturbate nearly, but not quite, to orgasm about an hour beforehand to increase prostate secretion. If his semen tastes bad, try altering his diet, and if that makes no difference, get a checkup — it can indicate health problems. She may like to know that an average ejaculation delivers about five calories and a dose of vitamin C.

skin

This is our chief extragenital sexual organ — underrated by men, who concentrate on the penis and clitoris; better understood by women. She says: "The smell and feel of a man's skin probably has more to do with sexual attraction (or the opposite) than any other single feature, even though you may not be conscious of it."

Skin stimulation is a major component of all sex. Not only its feel when touched, but its coolness, texture, and tightness are triggers for a whole range of sexual feelings. Built in; the so-called erogenous zones are the ones most rich in nerve endings — lips, earlobes, feet, buttocks, breasts as well as genitals. Sensitivity will vary — for both according to mood and for her according to menstrual cycle. But it can be boosted in some people by emphasis, and by adding other textures, especially fur, rubber, leather, or tight clothing. Much underrated part of human sexual response, to be played to the full if it turns you on (*see* friction rub, pages 112–13, *pattes d'araignée*, page 110, and tongue bath, page 120 — use these to educate your own and your partner's skin).

skin
its coolness, texture, and
tightness are triggers for a
whole range of sexual feelings

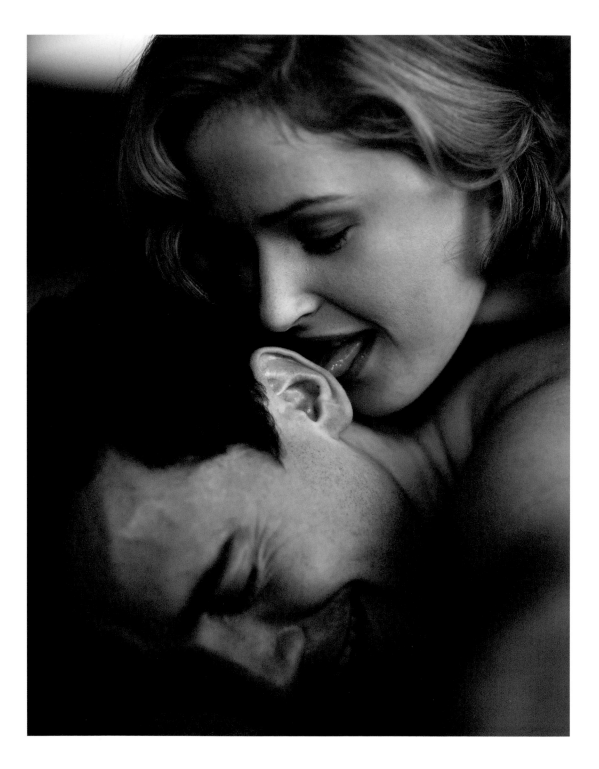

lubrication

Most natural lubrication comes from her — the male equivalent kicks in only just before orgasm, which is far too late. The normal excited vagina is correctly set for friction; if she is too wet, dry gently with a handkerchief-wrapped finger (not tissues — you will never stop finding the bits). But don't try to de-lubricate with lotions or potions; they can lacerate the vagina.

If she is too dry — it's normal for many women — it's likely because she is not sufficiently aroused; simply take the time and put in the effort. More lasting dryness can be due to stress, infections, medication, depression, hormonal ups and downs, and some medical conditions; see a doctor.

If more lubrication is needed, saliva is the best natural one. There is also much to be said for the many commercial possibilities offering added sensation, smells, and tastes, though note that oil-based ones destroy latex condoms, silicone-based ones destroy silicone sex toys, and some anesthetize. Be particularly sure to use lubricant if he is penetrating anywhere that doesn't naturally oblige — breasts, armpit, anus.

earlobes

Underrated erogenous zone, together with the adjacent neck skin — the small area behind the ear has an arousal hotline via the vagus nerve — and the nape of the neck. As with all extragenital sites, they are more responsive in women than men, whose skin is literally as well as metaphorically thicker. Once made sensitive (gentle fingering, sucking, and so on during build-up and before orgasm, to condition the response), earlobes can trigger full climax from manipulation alone. Be warned that some women find the noise of heavy breathing excruciating and a definite turnoff, so be careful (*see* blowing, page 121).

Heavy earrings help, and can actually maintain subliminal erotic excitement, especially if they are long enough to brush the neck when she turns her head — this is, in fact, the original function of the large Eastern and Spanish candelabra-type earrings.

Swinging weights as erotic stimuli to condition a particular area aren't confined to the ears. Safe installation and skillful handling of other types of body jewelry can provide additional erotic pleasure.

earlobes
can trigger full climax
from manipulation alone

navel
merits careful attention when
you kiss or touch

navel

Fascinating to lovers, like all the details of the human body. It's not only decorative but has a lot of cultivable sexual sensation; it fits the finger, tongue, glans, or big toe, and merits careful attention when you kiss or touch. Intercourse in the navel is practicable (there are stories of naive couples who thought that was the usual way, and it's a common childhood fantasy about how sex is conducted). If she is plump, she can hold up the skin on each side to make labia. In any case, the finger or tongue tip slips into it naturally in both sexes.

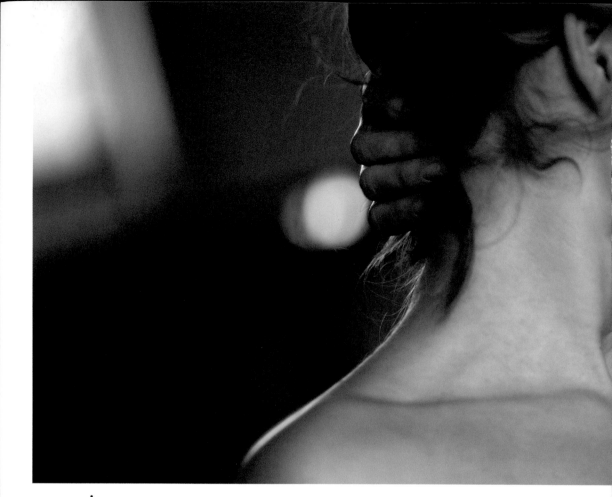

armpit

Classical site for kisses and can be used instead of the palm to silence your partner at climax – if you do use your palm, rub it over your own and your partner's armpit area first. Also a key site for pheromones, which cling, following perspiration, to underarm hair and generate arousal (*see cassolette*, pages 43–5). Which is why the original version of this book instructed that underarm hair should "on no account be shaved" – nowadays, depilation is more or less universal for her and not unknown for him; tastes change.

Axillary intercourse is an occasional variation. Handle it as for intermammary intercourse (*see* breasts, page 50), but with his penis under her right arm – well under, so that friction is on the shaft, not the glans, as in any other unlubricated area. Her left arm goes around his neck and he holds her right hand behind her with his right hand. She will get her sensations from the pressure against her breasts, helped by his big toe pressed to her clitoris if she wants it (*see* big toe, page 71). Not an outstandingly rewarding trick, but worth trying if you like the idea.

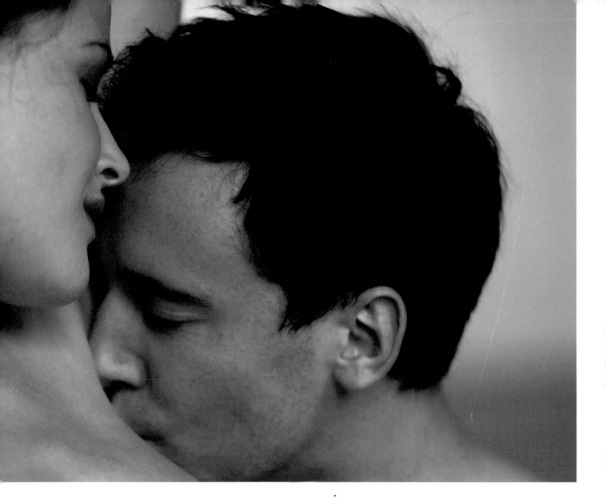

armpit
classical site for kisses

feet

Very attractive sexually to some people — he is able to get an orgasm, if he wishes, between the soles of her feet. Their erotic sensitivity varies a lot. Sometimes, when they are the only part you can reach, they serve as channels of communication, and the big toe makes a good penis substitute (*see* big toe, page 71). Tickling the soles excites some people out of their minds; for others it's agony, but increases general arousal. You can try it as a stimulus or, briefly, for testing the effectiveness of bondage (*see ligottage*, pages 252–3, and rope work, page 256). Firm pressure on the sole at the instep, however administered, is erogenous to most people. But so can almost any touch be in a woman who is that way minded — one can get a full orgasm from a foot, a finger, or an earlobe. Men respond far less but equally easily if the handling is skillful.

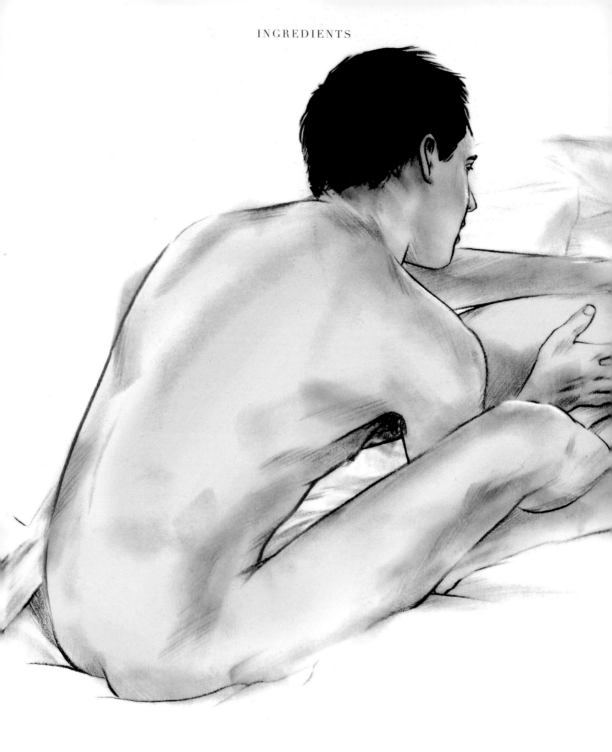

big toe
a magnificent erotic instrument

big toe

The pad of the male big toe applied to the clitoris or the vulva generally is a magnificent erotic instrument. The famous gentleman in erotic prints who is keeping six women successfully occupied is using tongue, penis, both hands, and both big toes. The toe can be used in mammary or armpit intercourse or any time he is astride her, or sits facing as she lies or sits. Make sure the nail isn't sharp. In a restaurant, one can surreptitiously remove a shoe and sock, reach out, and keep her in almost continuous orgasm with all four hands fully in view on the table top and no sign of contact – a party trick that rates as really advanced sex, though she may appear more than a little distracted. She has less scope, but can learn to masturbate him with his penis held between her two big toes. The toes reputedly have a direct nerve link to the genitals, and can be kissed, sucked, tickled, or tied with stimulating results.

hair

Head hair has a lot of Freudian overtones: in ancient mythology it's a sign of virility – witness Samson or Hercules – and some of these sexual associations have persisted to the present. Our culture, having learned in the past to associate long hair with women and short hair with manly conformity, has been occasionally excited to frenzy when young males rejected the stereotype and wore their hair long. Freud thought long female hair acted as reassurance to the male by being a substitute for the phallus that women don't have. Be that as it may, long male hair today tends to go with a less anxious idea of maleness.

Sex play with long hair is great because of its texture – you can handle it, touch each other with it, and generally use it as one more resource. Unless part of mutual mock fights, tugging and pulling is a total turnoff and will break you out of your sex trance. Long hair or a plait can be rolled to make a vagina substitute, or the penis lassoed with a loop of it, though some may object because it's a bore to wash.

Some women are turned on by a fair amount of masculine body hair because it looks virile, others are turned off by it because it looks animal – this seems to be a matter of attitude.

Male facial hair is another focus of convention – sometimes everyone has it as a social necessity or a response to convention, at other times it is persecuted, or confined to sailors, pioneers, and creative people such as artists and chefs. Nineteenth-century German philosopher Arthur Schopenhauer disapproved on the grounds that it was immodest to wear a sex signal in the middle of one's face. Today you can please yourself, or better, your partner.

pubic hair

Shave it off if you prefer: some people do. If you do shave it once, you are, however, committed to a prickly interregnum while it regrows. Some nowadays prefer it off in the interest of fashion or total nudity, or prefer the hardness of the bare pubis.

Others find it decorative and regard it as a resource. Try brushing it lightly and learn to caress with it – it can be combed, twirled, kissed, held, even pulled. In the woman it can move the whole pubis, skillfully handled, to the point of orgasm.

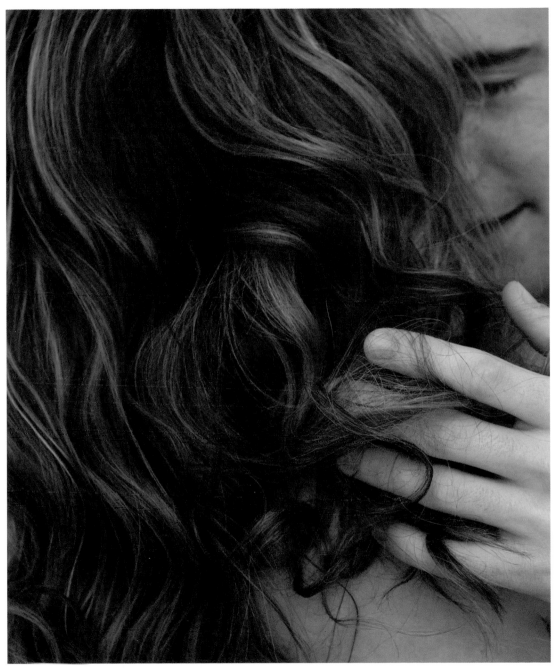

hair
handle it, touch each other with it

As a halfway house, she can trim it creatively, confining the triangle to the middle of the pubis with a bare strip each side – Brazilian style – removing hair that comes outside a G-string or a swimsuit, or trimming enough to make the vulva fully visible.

One myth that has proved remarkably persistent is that you can tell whether a blonde is natural from the color of her pubic hair. In reality, it's often several shades darker than head hair – consequently, in black-haired women it can be nearly blue.

Men can shave if they like, or if their partners like, but it's difficult to shave the scrotum. He may need to shave the penile shaft and root to use condoms – otherwise the hairs can get caught. This can produce sharp pain at a time when he should be experiencing intense pleasure.

health

We wish society would respect the link between this and sexuality. To us it's self-evident – despite all the cultural, religious, or simply anxiety-based hang-ups people have about keeping sex in its rightful place, whatever that is – that good health is supported by a good love life. Everyone, ill or well, deserves sex if they want it. To presuppose that illness or disability removes that wanting is to categorize sex in purely physical terms, to deny that it's there for affection, support, love – and moreover, to ignore the fact that it's a fundamental human need.

Yes, bad health can all too easily undermine sexual desire – even a heavy dose of the common cold can push sex right to the bottom of the list. One should never pressure oneself, or pressure one's partner, if suffering from illness. Longer term, it's not only pain or lack of function that hinders but also vulnerability and low self-esteem, particularly if illness directly affects sexual parts. You may feel so needy and dependent that sex seems a burden; you may feel so furious at your own ill health (or your partner's good health) that intimacy seems inappropriate. What you don't need is those around you adding to your problem by assuming you have lost – or never had – desire. To be human is to be at least potentially sexual, but there are some clinicians who suppose the young ill don't need sex education and the adult ill never need sex.

Both suppositions are wrong. Loving sex is everyone's right – alone if they have no partner. Anyone who can think about sex can experience desire. Anyone who can feel anything in mouth, breasts, clitoris, penis – or can fantasize about feeling – has at least potential for arousal. Anyone who can move fingers, tongue, or toes – or relate their fantasy – can arouse their partner. If none of that is possible or simply not wanted, then hugs, kisses, and hand-holding will give a sense of connection that can often do much to offset the absence of sex.

Knowledge is power, so get as much information as you can about what's possible for you (or for your partner if it's they who are ill) – *see* resources, pages 276–91. What feels good may not be what felt good before illness struck. Don't panic if your condition has affected genitals – brains can fill in the missing sensations; it's reckoned that over half of women with spinal-cord injury can orgasm with hand or mouth work.

Be practical and proactive here – joining a self-help group for the relevant disease or disability will give encouragement and support – and work with what you have, not what you don't have. If tiredness is an issue, make love just after waking; if pain or stiffness is an issue, take painkillers and a hot bath half an hour beforehand. Choose positions that take weight off vulnerable body parts – she can be taken from behind if she can't bear his weight and he can have her on top if he can't thrust. If erection is difficult, don't assume that's the way things have to be until you have explored the "little blue pill" possibility. And in any case, don't assume that intercourse is the gold standard – if hand, mouth, and a vibrator do the job, so be it. If desire is low or orgasm is challenging, check medications; some act to undermine sexual response but can be changed, given the right conversation with your doctor.

If hospitalized or institutionalized, you should ask for – if necessary, demand – privacy. If you are alone or both partners have limited mobility, some care workers are willing to assist, unbuttoning clothing, positioning limbs, and cleaning up afterwards, though it will need careful negotiation.

If you are hesitating to even mention the issue to health professionals, remember that they will have heard the "Can I have sex?" question many times before. If you don't trust your health professional – or he or she is erotophobic (some are) – then they can't help you, and you ought to change professionals. If the doctor actively prescribes no sex, challenge that opinion. If the answer really is no, only accept it if you are sure the doctor knows how much passion means to you; a good clinician will realize that stopping sex for any length of time is undermining. It bears repeating; for most people, good health is sustained by, and bad health improved by, a loving and regular sex life.

age

The only thing age has to do with sexual performance is that the longer you love, the more you learn. Young people (and some older ones) are firmly convinced that no one over fifty makes love, and it would be pretty obscene if they did. Ours isn't the first generation to know otherwise, but probably the first one that hasn't been brainwashed into being ashamed to admit it. No one need lose either sexual needs or sexual function with age; on the contrary, the best may be yet to come.

For women, the end of ovulation means the end of fertility, and for some this subtly affects their self-esteem. For others it represents a total liberation from contraceptive worry, and this, in addition to more sexual knowledge and a flurry of hormonal changes, can find her at a certain age slightly taken aback at her own high level of lust; remember too that a woman's ability to climax rises over the years.

As to menopausal symptoms, there is much debate right now about HRT (hormone replacement therapy); the jury is out and the best advice is to make an informed decision following regular talks with a clinician. If the evidence is against, there are medical or natural health solutions for the short-term problems of night sweats, hot flashes, and vaginal dryness, and the long-term risks of heart problems and bone-density reduction. Sex — with a partner or alone — will always help.

Men, who don't have as dramatic a physical change, may still both suffer disease and undergo an emotional "male menopause," which coincides with realizing that they haven't done what they fantasized about in youth, and that they had better do it now. This can lead to injudicious thrashing about, or simply a reassessment of their aims and opportunities very like a second adolescence. Women are increasingly hitting this too — the empty nest for both can be an intimation of mortality that in itself kick-starts a bout of midlife wet dreams.

Physically, the important changes for men over the first seven decades are that spontaneous erection occurs less often (a complete lack of erection is likely to be caused by ill health and should trigger an immediate doctor's visit); ejaculation takes longer to happen, which can be an advantage; and coital frequency tends to fall. It's a good idea not to try for ejaculation every time, which will give more mileage and no less mutual pleasure. But given a supportive and receptive partner, decent general health, and an absence of the belief that one ought to run out of steam, active sex lasts as long as life.

If activity is low and you are both happy with that, fine; sex is not compulsory. But about half of all couples over the age of sixty-five make love on a regular basis — a higher percentage, incidentally, than when the first edition of this book appeared more than 35 years ago – and many of the others will have stopped because of physical or relationship fragility, not sexual problems per se. The things that stop you from having sex with age are exactly the same as those that stop you from riding a bicycle (bad health, thinking it looks silly, no bicycle). The difference is that these things happen later for sex than for bicycles. So don't buy into the myth of age-limited performance – in any case, it's often culturally based; 90 percent of French women of a certain age think sex is important, as compared with only 30 percent of their British counterparts. *Vive la France!*

The most important thing is never to drop sex for any long period – if you do, you may have trouble restarting. Keep yourself going solo if you don't, for the time being, have a partner. What helps at this point: having sex in the morning when his testosterone levels are highest; making sure to keep a tube of lubricant handy for her vaginal dryness; her taking the lead and helping out with hand and mouth; him realizing that his hand and mouth may be just as acceptable as his penis; an easy ability on both sides to be experimental and broaden the repertoire.

Two warnings. Don't stop using contraception until she has been period-free for two years (if under fifty) or one year (over fifty). Moreover, don't stop using protection if there is any doubt at all about sexual history – a sixty year-old partner is actually more of a threat than a twenty-year-old because they are likely to have had a lot more experience (*see* safe sex, pages 96–8, and birth control, pages 144–5).

But those warnings aside, the older you are, the more potential you have for true intimacy – the sort that's not just based on hormonal surges but on a capacity to let go of your own insecurities and so deeply desire the other person. More confident, more knowledgeable, more experienced, you know what goes where and what to do with it; you know what works for you; you know what works for each other or – if you are newly come together – you know how to find out. Age brings patience and kindness, and an increased ability to both give and take; sex becomes more important, not less, as time goes on. As with so many things, later life is the time when you have tried everything and settle down to the things you like most – together. Some of the most spectacular and joyful sex imaginable is happening, right now, between people who would count themselves part of the "older generation."

sex maps

We are all born sexual beings; fetuses have erections, and from the age of a few months infants touch their genitals. We don't, however, grow up to become the same sexual beings: John Money's term "love map" – a mind template of the perfect lover – could be renamed "sex map," and everyone's sex map is different. Through early messages, through emotional events, through partner experiences, and through our culture's rites of passage, we all end up with a unique idea of what a sexual partner should do and what the sex act should involve. We all know, instinctively, what compels us and what repels us. We all know what our fetishes are.

On one level this matters not a bit. An individual sex map doesn't – or shouldn't – influence one's own self-value or a partner's opinion; it's unimportant whether one can swing from the chandeliers or not, whether one has had a queue of sexual partners or is a virgin.

On another level it matters enormously because sex maps underpin what we do and how we respond. They can get distorted; we may end up believing that all men get instantly hard on demand when they don't; that good sex just happens spontaneously when it doesn't. Plus, sex maps are often out of our awareness – we can fail to realize that we have unrealistic or unhelpful expectations, and so be doomed to disappointment. "Sex," as actor Shirley MacLaine once said, "is hardly ever just about sex."

The answer to all this is knowledge. It's never too late in life to find out just what sex is about for you. It's also never too early in a relationship to get to know a partner's expectations. Exploring each other's sex maps is highly advisable for any erotic liaison and an absolute necessity for anything that's going to last beyond the first night. Likes, dislikes, hates, fears, prejudices, and dreams: don't presume that a partner will know yours unless you tell them; don't presume you know theirs unless they have told you. Unpick them all, together, without feeling threatened, to appreciate as well as to understand – your own, revealed in comparison, as well as theirs.

Knowledge, it should be added, is important in other ways – it informs, improves, and optimizes the maps of young people growing up. We now know, through competent research, that sex education actively raises the age at which adolescents first have sex and lowers the number of partners they have and the number of risks they take; there is no excuse for withholding from children knowledge not only of the mechanics but also the underlying and informing emotions. To quote the first edition of this book: "Good sex education starts with respecting your children's modesty, answering their questions, and letting them see that you regard this as a topic for pleasurable interest, naturalness – and privacy, not secrecy."

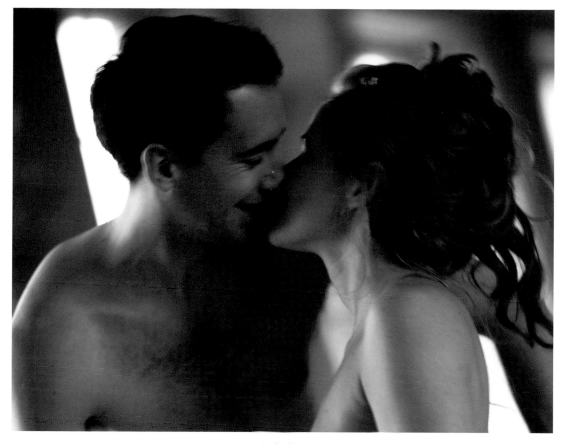

fidelity

people have to find their own fidelities

fidelity

Fidelity, infidelity, jealousy, and so on. We have deliberately not gone into the ethics of lifestyle. The facts are that few of us go through life with sexual experience confined to one partner only, infidelity figures increase year after year, and many people run multiple relationships on parallel tracks. See the five-to-seven early evening infidelity slot or the rich man's love nest. Yet most of us still remain monogamous in our long-term relationships, at least unless things start to go sour.

Don't buy into the myth that men do the betraying and women are immune — the female is just as programmed to stray, and if her statistics are lower, it's due to lack of opportunity, not instinct. (Besides, surveys usually measure lustful activity, whereas women's temptation is to fall in love, though the results can be even more devastating – think of *Anna Karenina*.)

There are as many reasons for infidelity as there are people, but in general for her it's a switching of loyalty when a central relationship disappoints; for him it's a boost to self-esteem when a central relationship invalidates. All this can be vice versa. Not to advocate, but this may be because humans have three sets of needs – for sex, romance, and deep attachment – and aren't always able to meet them all, long term, with one partner.

Whatever the temptations, however, fidelity is not only a good ideal but a good idea. We are more able to love – and to make love – if we are neither lying nor being lied to. Active deception always hurts a relationship. Complete frankness that is aimed to avoid guilt, or as an act of aggression against a partner, can do the same. The real problem arises from the fact that sexual relations can be anything, for different people and on different occasions, from a game to a total fusion of identities; the heartaches arise when each partner sees it differently.

There is no easy answer here. There is no sexual relationship that doesn't involve responsibility, because there are two or more people involved: anything that, as it were, militantly excludes a partner is hurtful, yet to be whole people we have at some point to avoid total fusion with each other – "I am I and you are you, and neither of us is on Earth to live up to the other's expectations." People who communicate sexually have to find their own fidelities. All we can suggest is that you discuss them, so that at least you know where each of you stands.

A final word on jealousy. Never play "get-even" games by flirting and worse. It may bring an errant partner to heel short term, but long term it's the worst kind of unloving behavior – and pointless; a relationship that doesn't hold together without such manipulations is not worth having. If you are prone to jealousy, particularly the desperately insecure, low-self-esteem kind, get counseling. If your partner is prone to betrayal, get out.

compatibility

Not whether you are "in love" or have chemistry, but whether – when you settle in for the long haul – the jigsaw puzzle pieces fit. If they do, then no external force will shake you; if they don't, however good you feel there will always be a sense of something missing. This is about having the same values, aims, goals – one reason why arranged (not forced) marriages often work better than the hearts-and-flowers variety. Two people see the world the same way, and that leaves them not so much focused on each other as, in French novelist and aviator Antoine de Saint-Exupéry's words, "looking together in the same direction" – as neat a definition of lasting love as one could hope to find.

Sexually, looking in the same direction is initially about complementary sexual preferences; if she fancies him and he also fancies him, then forget it, at least in bed. It's also about how important sex is; what's acceptable (erotica, infidelity, fetishes, and so on); how much and how often. Similarity not quantity matters here – they can both be happy with it once a year and hence be happy with each other. Get the match on these right and the connection will be bone deep.

Sexual incompatibilities that surface once the first rush of love is over are mostly due to loss of love, not lust. But keep the sexual fit and it will be much harder to fall out of love; this may seem like kindergarten stuff, but in and of itself, passion will act as a safeguard for the whole relationship. Properly done, sex is not only based on compatibility; it also creates it.

desire

What prompts desire at first is insecurity. We are unsure of the other's response, unsure of the ending to the story; the possibility that we might not get what we want creates a kind of obsessive focus. Thus medieval "courtly love," thus psychologist Dorothy Tennov's "limerence," thus *Romeo and Juliet* and most of the lyrics of contemporary music. When and if consummation comes, we are left with an air of astonished gratitude.

For desire to grow, what's needed after that is mutual appreciation. One doesn't necessarily need commitment – society is now past the point where a woman only allowed herself to lust once she had the ring on her finger – but believing that the person we desire is still going to desire us in the morning lowers our emotional barriers and lets us get serious about the business of wanting. What then develops is everything this book is about.

If desire fails early on, it's probably because sometimes once we have what we want, we don't want it anymore, and the most sensible thing for both parties at that point is to let the whole thing go. Once love is established, however, a temporary dip shouldn't be cause for panic, withdrawal, or infidelity; no one, male or female, can enjoy sex when one is dead with fatigue, when one has just given birth, when children are hammering on the door, or in the middle of a busy street. If desire fails totally and permanently, the likely culprits are medical or hormonal problems, depression, or relation-

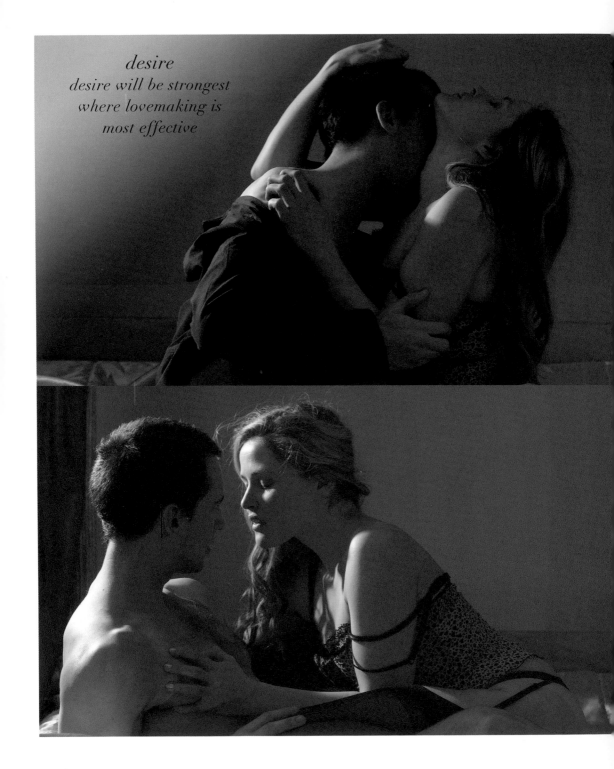

desire
desire will be strongest
where lovemaking is
most effective

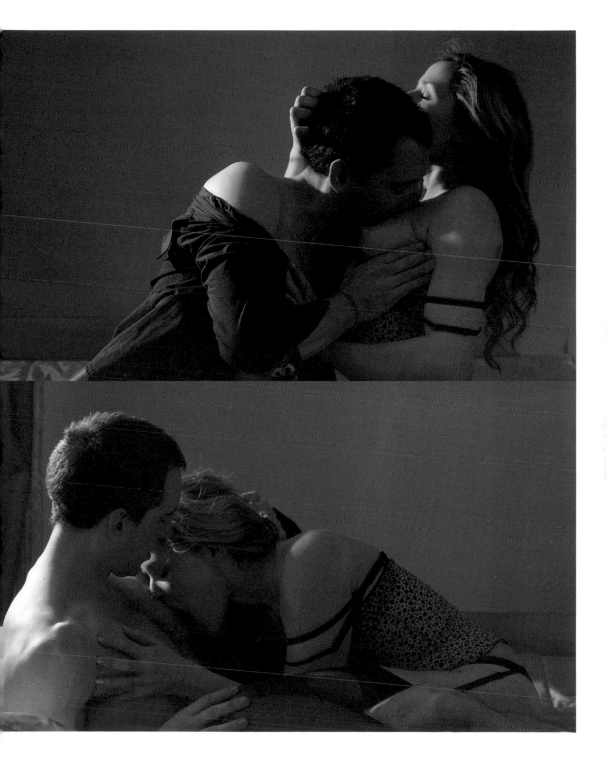

ship crisis – and it's not disloyal but sensible to rush off to the doctor or the relationships counselor (*see* resources, page 278–81). Ignoring the problem and teeth-gritting – following Alice, Lady Hillingdon's advice to "lie back and think of England" – will simply make the problem worse as the lack of pleasure gradually seeps into your blood. Eventually, all that will be left is negative reaction; a partner's touch becomes something to shrink from. Get help now.

Other than these situations, a strong and lasting desire for each other is a reasonable request to make of the love gods, but serious players know that the gods help those who help themselves. Desire will be strongest where lovemaking is most effective; that means both partners should know how to arouse creatively and bring the other to climax as a matter of course, however much teach-and-learn it took to get there. In the end, Pavlov's dogs stopped salivating when no food appeared; it's wise to make sure that most meals satisfy both diners at least most of the time.

Intense desire is not just about passion, however, but also about emotion – one reason why the title of this book contains words referring to both. If we are to keep lusting, we need to keep feeling; if resentment and irritation lead to emotional anesthetization, that will inevitably lead to physiological anesthetization and a total shutdown of sensation experience. This is not to say that feelings have to be positive all the time – even the best of relationships contain some of what sex therapist David Schnarch describes as "reptilian" reactions; that is, going in for the kill. But to keep on feeling passion, you need to have the courage to keep feeling full stop. Rage if you have to, but don't disengage.

Remember that desire will be strongest in situations where it's awarded the most space and encouragement; if you want each other, act on it. A truly dedicated lover works at their art, and realizes that art is no less valuable for having to be worked at. The more sex one has, the more one will want – even with his biological limiter, that is true for him, and it's even more true for her.

love

We use the same word for man-woman, mother-child, child-parent, and other interpersonal relations – rightly, because they are a continuous spectrum. In talking about sexual relations, it seems right to apply it to any relationship in which there is mutual tenderness, respect, and consideration – from a total interdependence where the death of one partner maims the other for years, to an agreeable night together. The intergrades are all love, all worthy, all part of human experience.

Some meet the needs of one person, some of another – or of the same person at different times. That's really the big problem of sexual ethics, and it's basically a problem of self-understanding, and of communication. You can't assume that your "conditions of love" are applicable to, or accepted by, any other party; you can't assume that these won't be changed quite unpredictably in both of you by the experience of loving; you can't necessarily know your own mind.

If you are going to love, these are risks you have to take, and don't depend simply on whether or not you have sex together – though that is such a potentially overwhelming experience that tradition is right in pinpointing it. Sometimes two people know each other very well, or think they have worked things out through discussion, and they may be right. But even so, if it's dignifiable by the name of love, it's potentially an open-ended experience. Tradition has tried to cut the casualties by laying down all kinds of schedules of morality, but these never work 100 percent in practice. Nor are they of much use in classifying the merits of different kinds of relationships (*see* fidelity, page 79).

If sexual love can be – and it is – the supreme human experience, it must be also a bit hazardous. It can give us our best and our worst moments. In this respect it's like mountain climbing – over-timid people miss the whole experience; reasonably balanced and hardy people accept the risks for the rewards, but realize that there's a difference between this and being fool-hardy. Love, moreover, involves someone else's neck besides your own. At least you can make as sure as may be that you don't exploit or injure someone – you don't take a novice climbing and abandon them halfway up when things get difficult. Getting them to sign a consent form before they start isn't an answer either. There was a great deal to be said for the Victorian idea of not being a cad ("person devoid of finer or gentlemanly feelings"). A cad can be of either sex.

When this book was first written, the world was in the middle of the most radical rethinking of sexuality ever – and the subsequent rethinking of love. The prediction then was that sex and love could be divorced, and no-strings sex is certainly now more common. But most of us still require a connection before we can do any more than simply perform; love may not be all you need, but it's an essential for any except the most basic satisfaction. Equally, when the going gets rough in relationships, good, pleasurable sex can bring you through. When you make love, you do exactly that.

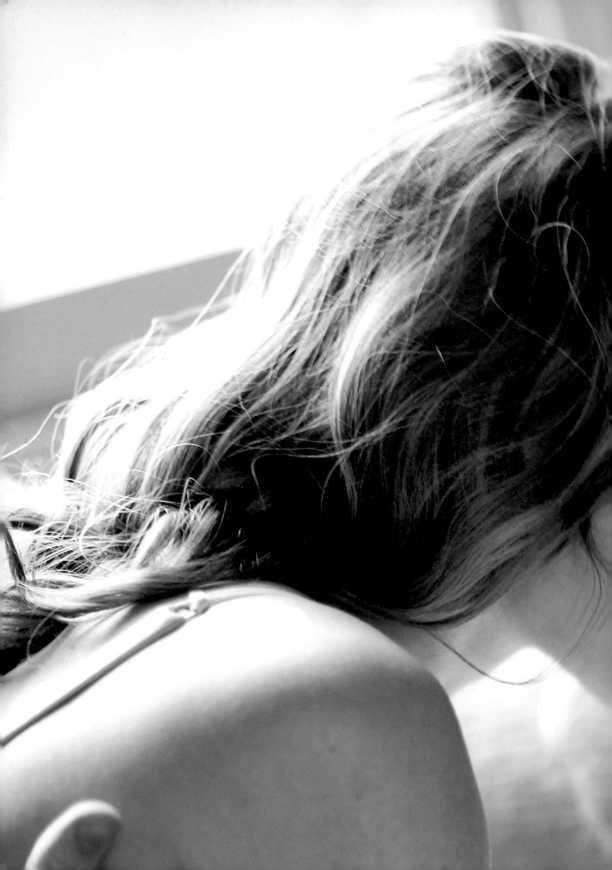

appetizers

real sex

The sort our culture and most mass-media propaganda don't recognize: not that intercourse, or masturbation, or genital kisses aren't real sex, but some other things are real sex too, which people need, but that don't excite our time and age. We can list some: being together in a situation of pleasure, or of danger, or just of rest; touching, even if that doesn't involve any of the traditionally erotic zones; old-fashioned expedients like holding hands (permissiveness makes for more orgasms, but we miss out on the simple

real sex
being together, touching, holding hands

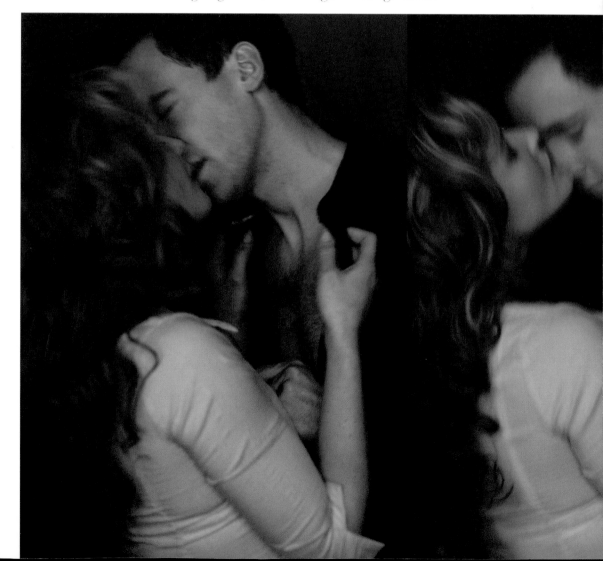

pleasures of looking, smiling, flirting, dating, kisses, and holding each other close — the bonding elements that vagina-obsessed males think of as schmaltz); sleeping together even without, or especially after, intercourse.

Most women know all this, but they are as shy about telling it to males, for fear of seeming over-sentimental, as males are about confiding object preferences or forceful needs. Don't get stuck with the view that only those things that Auntie calls sexual are sexual. In a book on sexual elaboration, this needs saying, if you are concerned with love rather than an Olympic pentathlon. People in our culture who are hung up on the Olympic bit don't get much from using the gentler options, unless over time such use builds the realization of just how important those options really are.

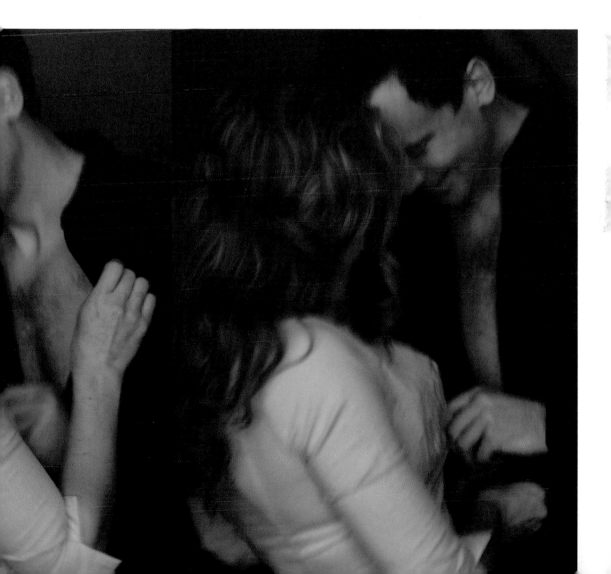

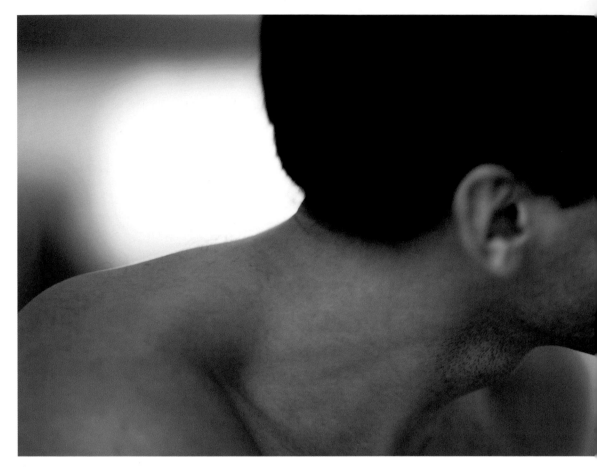

food

Dinner is a traditional preface to sex. In old-time France or Austria, one booked a restaurant room with no handle on the outside of the door. At the same time, there is a French saying that love and digestion went to bed together and the offspring was apoplexy. This isn't quite true. On the other hand, immediately after a heavy meal is not an ideal moment for sex — you can easily make your partner, especially the woman if she is underneath, sick.

A meal can be an entire erotic experience in itself — for a demonstration of how a woman can excite a man by eating a chicken leg or a pear "at" him, cannibal-style, see the lovely burlesque in the 1963 film *Tom Jones* or the outrageously sensuous equivalents in *Tampopo* and *9½ Weeks*.

A meal à deux is, quite certainly, a direct lead-in to love play (*see* big toe, page 71, and remote control, page 246), but don't overindulge on alcohol. Recent studies show it lowers inhibitions and increases euphoria, particu-

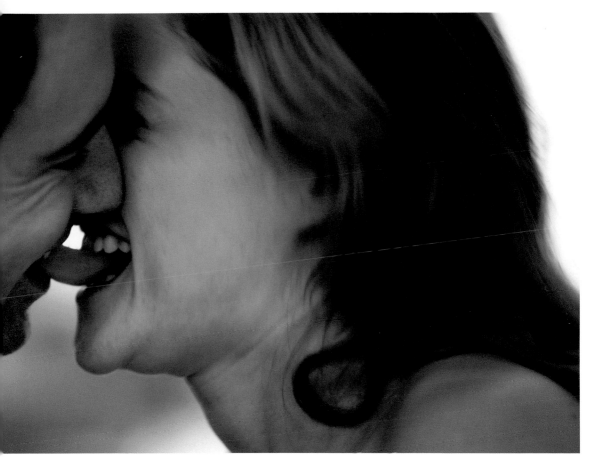

food
a meal can be an entire erotic experience in itself

larly for women, but is the most common cause of unexpected erectile problems. If you are serious about sex, develop a liking for mineral water.

Love and food mixed well in Greek and Roman times when you reclined together on a couch, or fed one another (geishas do this still). Some people enjoy food-and-sex games (ice cream on the skin, grapes in the pussy, and so on), which are great for regressive orality, but messy for an ordinary domestic setting; take care too with sugary foods, which can cause yeast infections, and oily foods, which can shred condoms. Most lovers with privacy like to eat naked together and take it from there.

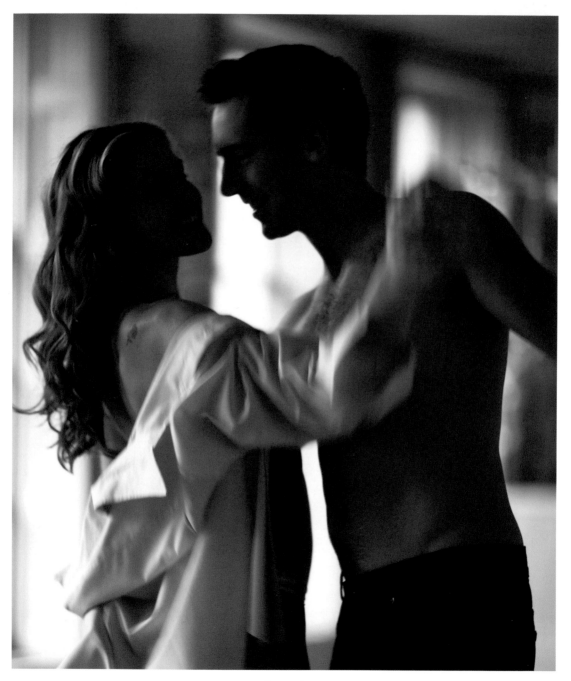

dancing
good lovers dance well together

dancing

All dancing in pairs looks towards intercourse. In this respect the Puritans were absolutely right. The development of no-contact dances has come about because one doesn't now need a social excuse to embrace, but as an excitant it need not involve contact at all – in fact, most dancing today is far more erotic than a clinch because you aren't too close to see one another. At its best, this sort of dance is simply intercourse by remote control (*see* remote control, page 246).

Most good lovers dance well together. You can do it publicly or in private, clothed or naked. Stripping one another while dancing is a sensation on its own. Don't hurry to full intercourse – dance until his erection is unbearable and she is almost coming, brought there by rhythm and the sight and perfume of each other alone. Even then you need not stop.

Most couples can insert and continue dancing, either in each other's arms or limbo-style, linked only by the penis, provided they are the appropriate heights. Unfortunately, this means that the woman needs to be at least as tall as the man, while as a rule she is going to be shorter. Otherwise, he has to bend his knees, which is tiring. If you can't dance inserted, and if she is small, pick her up into one of the Hindu standing positions, legs around waist, arms around neck, and continue in this way. If she is too heavy to pick up, you can turn her and take her stooping from behind, still keeping the dance going.

Seduction, or encouragement, while dancing is a natural. In the days of formal dancing, one wished that the woman had her breasts on her back, where one could reach them, but that would have made it too easy. Gentle pressure, rhythm, sight and scent, and a knowledge of remote-control methods are all that's needed to bring the dance on to its erotic conclusion.

femoral intercourse

Another dodge, like clothed intercourse (*see* pages 94–95), to preserve virginity, avoid pregnancy, and so on, used in past cultures that cared about virginity and had no contraceptives, or in present cultures that advise abstinence before marriage. Comes for us under the heading of substitutes.

Used from before or behind, or in any other posture where she can press her thighs together. The penis goes between them, with the shaft between her labia but the glans well clear of the vagina, and she presses hard. Gives the woman a special set of sensations – sometimes keener than on penetration, so worth trying. Given condoms and other forms of birth control, and safe sex, one need not be so rigid about technique as were our forefathers, who had to try to keep sperm out of the vagina at any cost. With care, one can do this from behind with the glans actually on the clitoris, with striking results. A good menstrual variant, useful if she is vaginally sore, or for at least a few strokes before he goes in as usual.

clothed intercourse

Really a heavy-petting technique: she keeps her panties or G-string on, he carries out all the movements of straight intercourse as far as the cloth will allow. Favorite ethnologic variant, chiefly for premarital intercourse. Apparently called *droogneuken* in Dutch, but oddly, many cultures have no special word for the practice.

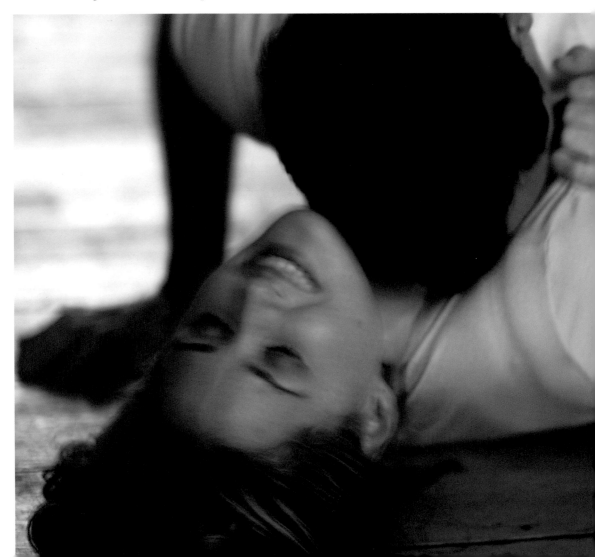

Not reliable as a contraceptive or protective unless the ejaculation position is fully interfemoral; that is, with the glans well clear of the vulva, cloth or no cloth. Some people like this either as a starter or during menstrual periods. Inclined to be "dry" and make the man sore if it goes on too long or involves starched material of the sort denim jeans are made – go gently. Many women can get a fair orgasm from it.

clothed intercourse
all the movements of straight intercourse

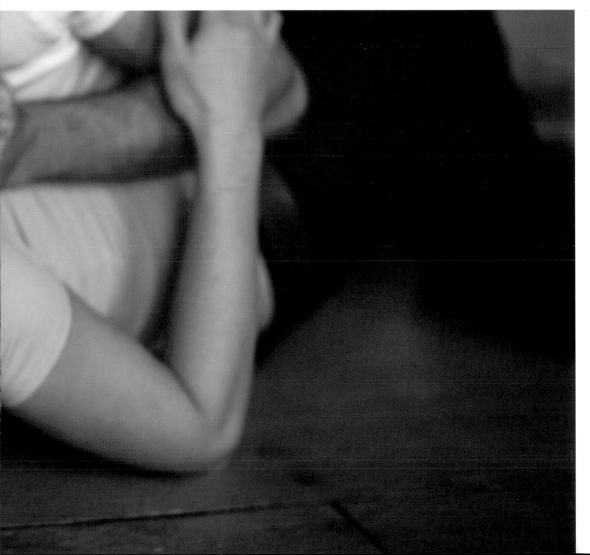

safe sex

We are, thankfully, past the point where HIV is an automatic death sentence. However, in some parts of the world it still is a death sentence, and worldwide, sexually transmitted diseases (STDs) are at an all-time high. This is no time to be careless.

The threats are many. Gonorrhea and syphilis are still with us, and the former is getting harder to eradicate because of resistant strains. Plus herpes, trichomoniasis, bacterial vaginosis, thrush, viral hepatitis, crabs, scabies, HIV of course, the human papilloma (wart) virus, and chlamydia. We now know that the wart virus triggers a majority of cases of cervical cancer, while chlamydia can cause infertility (*see* resources, pages 276–91). For all these reasons, here are the guidelines.

- Whatever your age, sex, or sexual experience, you could be at risk. Once it became apparent that AIDS was not going to decimate the developed world (and despite the fact that it's still decimating the developing world), there was an arrogant conviction that protection was optional. Wrong; each day over a million people worldwide catch an STD. Also wrong is that STDs are solely the problem of the young and sexually active, who are, in fact, often informed and careful; older lovers – freshly divorced and convinced that they and their cohort are safe – are often not.

- Risk comes from exchange of body fluids, so think about saliva, blood, urine, and feces as well as semen and vaginal fluids. Penetration is key, but a scratch or bite that breaks the skin surface is also dangerous, as is oral sex. Yes, oral sex – it's the risk factor that everyone ignores because licking your lover through a condom seems so prissy, but infection is more than possible, and women are particularly at risk.

- One's main reassurances are the condom (male and female), the dam, and the medical glove – used for intercourse, anal sex, sex toys, and oral sex. Let's not pretend latex improves lovemaking; but sometimes you simply have to do what's needed.

- You probably know the drill, but let's revise condom care: store away from sunlight; don't keep past the sell-by date; use a new one for every intercourse; check for rips and tears; have the condom in place from the start to the end of sexual contact; if it splits, get emergency contraception. Above all, follow the World War II British army motto: "Put it on before you put it in."

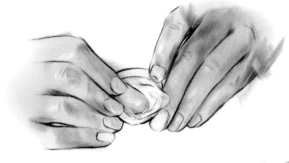

1 To use a condom, carefully remove it from the foil packet and check it is the right way round, ready to roll down.

2 Squeeze the end of the condom between forefinger and thumb and place it over his erect penis.

3 Use your other hand to unroll the condom gently down. Keep squeezing the end between forefinger and thumb.

4 Make sure the condom is rolled down the full length of the penis.

- The condom test is a good way of knowing whether you have found a decent, sensible partner. If your newly found love won't use protection, you are in bed with a witless, irresponsible, and uncaring person.

- When your newly found love has become a long-standing and committed love, the way forward is for both of you to get tested before having unprotected sex, and then to stay faithful. Is it unromantic to suggest testing? Yes, but it's also being realistic. Even if your partner has had only one other partner and that person has had only one other, and so on and on, you are still potentially linked with a host of unproven and unknown infections. If you love each other, testing is the best way of demonstrating that. If you don't love each other, even less reason to take things on trust.

- With sex toys used by non-long-term partners, slip a condom over before use, and between uses clean with antibacterial wipes or the sort of cleaning pads sold for the purpose in sex shops.

- Check yourselves regularly for anything unusual — itching, rashes, lumps, warts, discharge, fever, swollen glands, abdominal discomfort, and bleeding or pain during sex, urination, or defecation.

- Respond to symptoms by going for a checkup immediately. Sexual health clinic staff really have seen it all before. Most infections, if caught early, can be treated by antibiotics; the exceptions are herpes, some strains of hepatitis, and the HIV virus, which are for life (*see* resources, pages 276–91). If you have contracted an STD, or have put yourself at risk of doing so, tell your current partner and seek clinical advice about whether you need to tell former ones.

- Regular medical checkups are a good idea even if you are both faithful; some STDs can lie dormant. Plus, of course, you can never be entirely certain of fidelity.

phone sex

Not the pay-for, professional, chat-line type — which doesn't seem to fit in a book such as this — but loving arousal between two people who know each other's real names and real natures. The limitations — just sound, no visuals, no touch — can drive separated partners mad with frustration, but can also be its main attraction. The world goes away and all that remains is pure pleasure and two voices.

With only sound as feedback, one needs to tell more, describe fully, be ultra-clear about progress. Codes will develop that signal each one's shifts of mood or movement; rises of volume or breathing pace when speeding up, slowing down, starting to come; favored words and phrases that trigger memories or fantasies. Create a scenario; take it in turns to tell a story; ask intimate questions and answer them; make a confession of lust or love. For her in particular, fingers, vibrator, and sound will likely do it all; if he hankers for the visuals too, get her to do it in front of a mirror and describe herself (*see* mirrors, page 241).

Once supremely in sync, slide into control games. There is a special arousal in being directed long-distance — the other's voice alone telling one to "stop . . . start . . . pause" while one fights the temptation to tip over. And there is a special pleasure in knowing that your lover is being aroused solely by your direction, and is doing precisely what you instruct. If in charge, keep yourself simmering too, so that when the other is on the edge, you can first give them permission to "come now," then immediately join them in climax.

words

"For women . . . the G-spot is in the ears," said author Isabel Allende, but his blood too can be roused by the right tone. Mutual vocabulary is essential; tastes are highly individual, and largely non-negotiable, and what one may feel is arousing, the other may think is too crude, clinical, or aggressive.

With a new partner — or with an old partner but a new word — whisper and calibrate the response; if there is a flinch, don't use it again. If it's you who's flinching, say so and together work out an arousing alternative. There are more than 250 words for penis in the English language and 200 for clitoris; if none of these play, like the couple in *Lady Chatterley's Lover*, christen John Thomas and Lady Jane yourselves

If you aren't comfortable talking dirty but want to be, practice key phrases while you are self-pleasuring alone. If you aren't comfortable talking dirty and don't want to be, relax; there is no requirement.

technology

Has had a bad press, due to addiction, cyberaffairs, and so on. But don't blame the medium; its opportunities outweigh its problems, and in any case, whenever there is a new human development, it comes with down- as well as upsides. So long as you are not using the Internet as a bolt hole to escape real relationships, technology is a good idea for the same reasons that phone sex (*see* page 99) is: it offers a new take and new possibilities, and fills a need in a world where love can be forced to span oceans.

Obvious is that the Internet is a key resource for inspiration and ideas. There is a wealth of material out there: erotica, help lines, online counseling, and special-interest websites for every taste and a few undreamed of; particularly charming is the one that tells you how to make your own sex toys from melons, balloons, and empty bottles of washing-up liquid. Online coverage of sex is expanding so quickly that it would be pointless to attempt a listing; simply surf.

This is not a book about finding a sexual partner, so let's pass over Internet dating except to repeat the usual warnings about safety, which are these. However close one may feel to someone one has been chatting with online, treat them as one would any blind – unseen and unknown – date; that is, with care. Don't give out details; don't meet alone without safety nets; don't take it personally if, on meeting, there is no chemistry and they run off into the night. Reputable dating sites say all this in their guidelines – read, learn, and bear in mind that the nature of the Internet creates speedy yet false intimacy that may cloud your judgment.

Using new technology for erotic purposes, on the other hand, is the ultimate in safe sex – no exchange of body fluids involved. Text message, e-mail, webcams, teledildonics can all be used to wind each other up to fever pitch during the working day prior to extended evening action, to navigate more extended separations, and to play out dangerous or impractical fantasies without risk. For word-based text and e-mail, the key is in the description (where you are, what you are wearing, what you are doing to yourself, what you would like to do to the other). Don't be held back by fear of spelling and grammar – it's irrelevant and in any case too much control over the protocols of language can not only inhibit but come across online as just too manicured. Yet equally, don't aim to talk dirty – in black and white it can seem harsh or simply silly. Instead just say what's happening, moment by moment, what you are doing, imagining, wanting, above all, feeling.

Feedback may not be instant, so bridge the gaps between sending and receiving; she in particular has to learn to keep herself at pitch despite pauses until climax is imminent. Vibrators really come into their own here.

frequency

The right frequency for sex is as often as you both enjoy it. You can no more have "too much" sex than you can over-empty a toilet cistern (*see* excesses, page 201), though he can cut his short-term fertility by having too many ejaculations, and you don't want to make intercourse such an anxious business that you have to stick to a daily timetable. Two or three times a week is a statistical average; new couples have it much oftener, established couples typically less. Some people do stick to a pretty regular schedule – others like intensive weekends at intervals.

The people who stick strictly to coital orgasm are usually opting for fewer climaxes than those who mix coitus with oral, manual, and other plays, because these increase the number of climaxes most men can get in a session. You should devise your own mix, in the light of your own responses: if one partner needs more, the accessory methods are useful to supply their needs and match them to yours.

Frequency falls off normally with age (*see* age, pages 76–7) , but there is no age when you won't, on some special occasion, surprise yourself. Don't be compulsive about frequency and don't panic about surveys, which are often based on respondent exaggeration. Realize there will be times when one of you just doesn't feel like it – through preoccupation, fatigue, or a traumatized response to important life events like birth or death – and don't enforce a timetable on your partner or on yourself. If it's still not happening, check the physicals, medications, fatigue, stress, and so on, then wonder whether anger or resentment is the root cause. It isn't any kind of failure to ask for expert help (*see* resources, pages 276–91).

priorities

Not a problem when we start a relationship; everything gets moved aside in the name of sex. As we settle, it is sex that gets moved aside. The Kinsey Institute says that contemporary women have less sex than their 1950s counterparts because they have so little uncommitted time in their lives; a finding that would ring true for many.

Deciding to prioritize sex may be guilt-inducing; we don't want to compromise other commitments and put our pleasure before our duties. But actually, once one realizes that sex is not an indulgence but a necessity, it all becomes easier. Keep a diary and see what can be canceled or put on hold. Book in one night a week and one weekend a month. Don't aim to make love but just to talk, embrace, be together; sex will happen if it's meant to. Usually, given time and space, it is meant to.

Add children and the whole thing becomes both more difficult and more essential. Difficult because it's inconvenient to incorporate sex into family life, essential because it needs to happen in order to keep love fueled and the family together. Sex can't be put on hold until the children are grown; if it is, the relationship may walk out the door at about the same time as the offspring fly the nest – or worse, well before. So act now. With toddlers, who for safety reasons one can't simply ban from the bedroom, enforce an early bedtime and buy a baby monitor. With older children, fit a lock to the bedroom door and state clearly when you are uninterruptable. If caught in flagrante, stay calm – children will take their cue from your emotions, and if you are unembarrassed they will be untroubled. Alternatively, leave them with grandparents, friends, or sitters while you take serious and extended private time. Ignore any qualms here; sex will make you a better parent, not a worse one.

seduction

If used in the traditional definition of the word – "to entice someone into an act that they will probably regret" – not good. The ultimate seducer, Casanova, incidentally, was enticed, pressured, and forced just as much as he did the enticing, and not only regretted but sometimes actively resented his sexual liaisons.

If used to mean "to woo someone into sex when you both want it," much better; a validation manifested in the willingness to make the effort. Attention, compliment, clear intention, light touch, a drawing in and drawing on, the assumption that one person is willing to woo, and the other is worth the wooing; all this is in itself immensely persuasive.

In an established relationship, always at least try to respond to seduction. Men have less choice here – if they really don't want to, they often simply can't – but neither sex will be seducible in the context of a looming deadline or a screaming child, though both he and she can still offer affection and open arms. You should at least be willing to touch and kiss for a few minutes to see if your body will respond; it often does, even if you are convinced it's not going to. It should be added that it's not a partner's duty to have sex, nor their right to demand sex – and both sides should be willing to take no for an answer.

In a new or potential relationship, reacting to seductive moves is a different game. Rules vary from culture to culture, but a sound guideline is to say yes if you want to and, more important, if you are sure you will still be comfortable with the decision the morning after and when sober. Never say yes if you feel out of control (via alcohol, drugs, emotional blackmail), out of guilt or duty, or if you can't practice safe sex. If a new partner insists on physicality earlier than you want it, their pleasure is more important to them than your comfort and they are therefore not worthy of you. All this applies to him just as much as to her. Say a clear no and trust your instincts.

There are currently some charming websites on the Internet offering "seduction skills" that are really camouflaged training courses – usually for him – on how to be more socially competent, how to find out what a woman wants and then genuinely and affectionately deliver; the result of such training is likely to be an increased ability to commit and to make that commitment work. There are also some truly appalling websites for him and for her, and even some books, that talk of "victim" or "prey" and then suggest manipulations such as "make her feel insecure" or "don't call, make him sweat." This is abusive, whichever sex does it.

The Barefoot Doctor says, instead: "Humbly, confidently make your desires known to all relevant parties, then let go and wait." That would work well for most of us.

bathing

Bathing together is a natural concomitant of sex and a splendid overture or tailpiece. Taking an ordinary bath together has a charm of its own, though someone has to lean against the plumbing. Soaping one another all over (rinse off before penetration or risk allergies to the lather, particularly for her) and drying one another are "skin games" that lead naturally to better things; after intercourse, a bath together is a natural, gentle comeback to domesticity or work. There are now luxurious large baths and Jacuzzis on offer, as well as hot tubs for outside, year-round bathing entertainment.

Actual coitus is possible, and fun, in the shower if your heights match; a showerhead is often the only convenient point in most houses or hotels for attaching a partner's hands. Don't pull the fixture down, however – it isn't weight-bearing. Movable shower attachments also offer possibilities for water stimulation, but don't aim it forcibly into the vagina – water under pressure, like air, can do internal damage.

No ordinary domestic or hotel bath is big enough for intercourse without punishing your elbows. Besides the novelty, there isn't much point anyway. It's easier with her on top, and sex toys can be bought waterproof for use by the one outside the bath on the one in it.

Sex and outdoor bathing is a different matter, but check local customs and laws. The whole idea of intercourse in water is that it's like weightlessness or flying – a woman who is too big for all those Hindu climbing and standing postures becomes light enough to handle, and one can prop her at angles no acrobat could hold. Meanwhile, there is the sea, after dark, when it's warm enough – on a gradually shelving beach one can have enough privacy even by day, and even reemerge clothed: spectators will take it for lifesaving. A pool has extras like steps and useful handholds.

Water doesn't hinder friction, though its relative chill may mean that it takes some brisk rubbing to get an erection even in a very eager male. It might be a good idea to insert before going in, if possible, or for the woman to wear a diaphragm; seawater could trigger infections and chlorinated pool water might just possibly be an irritant, as it is to the eyes. You can have excellent straight intercourse lying in the surf if you can get a beach to yourselves, but sand is a problem, and keeps appearing for days afterwards. A floating mattress is effectively a water bed, but it's hard to stay on it without concentrating.

We have heard of people combining coitus with swimming, and even scuba diving, but they gave no practical details. Underwater coitus, if more than a token contact, would use up vast amounts of air because of the over-breathing that goes with orgasm.

Sadly, water sex isn't fundamentally safe sex; condoms can slip off or be affected by the water, heat, or chemicals, while spermicides may wash away and water-based lubricants simply dissolve. To enjoy any of the above approaches safely, you both need to be infection-free, contraceptively protected, and sure of your fellow bathers.

bathing
a splendid overture or tailpiece

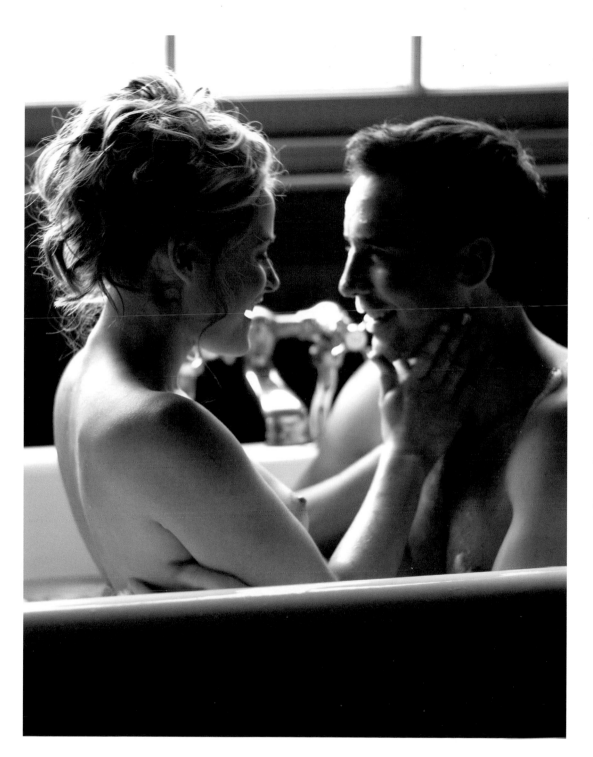

beds
take one another at
any hour of the night
and relax together
immediately afterwards

beds

Still the most important piece of domestic sexual equipment. Really enthusiastic sex usually involves, at one time or another, almost every piece of furniture in the house, at least experimentally, but the bed is its commonest venue. Most beds on the market are designed by people who think they are intended to sleep on. The problem arises from the fact that the ideal surface for most kinds of intercourse needs to be rather harder than is comfortable for a whole night's sleep. One solution is to have two beds, one for sex and the other for sleeping, but this is a counsel of affluence, and in any case the need to move disrupts the best part of the night – the total relaxation that follows complete love. Enormous or circular beds look suggestive, but have no real advantages over a full-size double bed.

There are a few points we would consider before giving a seal of approval. First, since one uses the sides as well as the surface, the height needs to be right. The top of the mattress should be exactly level with the man's pubic bone – then, if he puts her on or over it, she will be at the right height from in front or from behind. For some operations, especially bondage scenes if you like them, bedposts are essential, preferably tall ones, like those that hold up the canopies of antique beds, but not a footboard, as you may want to use the end of the bed for bending her over, backwards or forwards (*see ligottage*, pages 252–3, and rope work, pages 256–7). Massive old bed frames have great advantages in that they don't rattle or collapse. The mattress needs to be as hard as you can tolerate for comfortable sleep.

A double bed is essential; anything less forfeits the chief sexual joy of living and sleeping together – the fact that you can take one another at any hour of the night when both want it, and relax together immediately afterwards. If you have room, have a single bed as well, in case either partner is sick and feels more comfortable solo – twin beds have no place in a full sexual relationship.

Besides the bed itself, you need four pillows – two very hard to go under the buttocks, and two soft to sleep on. The room must be warm at all times of the year – warm enough to sleep without getting chilled, and without nightclothes if you wish. Duvets are generally better than blankets; they move with you as you move and don't restrict. Water beds, now reminiscent

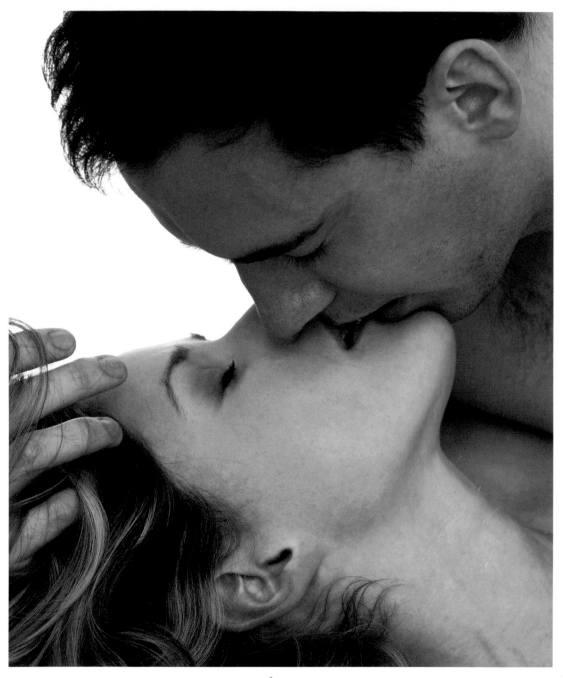

kisses
range from a mere touch to a second penetration

of glitzy glam and lava lamps, and only encountered rarely, nevertheless produce extraordinary sensations, and they have a natural period of resonance that tends to take over – one has to move in their rhythm, but this in itself is a stimulating constraint.

kisses

These, at one level, don't require teaching, but it's easy to be so set on insertion that one overlooks them (*see* real sex, pages 88–9). Lip and tongue kisses add immensely to lovemaking in all face-to-face positions. Breast kisses are essential if the woman isn't to miss a whole range of feeling, while genital kisses (*see* mouth work, pages 136–41) are a tender resource on their own. Kisses can be put anywhere on the body; they can be given with lips, tongue, penis, labia, or eyelashes – mouth kisses range from a mere touch to the kiss *à la cannibale*, which leaves a bruise.

A lot of people maintain mouth contact continuously throughout intercourse, and prefer face-to-face positions for this reason. The deep tongue kiss can either be a second penetration, the man's tongue imitating exactly the rhythm of what's going on elsewhere, or she can give it, penetrating him, to call the rhythm. Even without any penetration, some people favor a tongue battle, which can last minutes or even hours, bringing several orgasms for the woman; this form of non-genital heavy petting is called *maraîchignage*. If you are in private, move on to breasts, and go from there.

Another pleasure is to make her a carpet of flowers, by covering every inch of her body with small, close kisses: then she can reply, using lipstick to mark where she has been. From there it's only a little way to doing the same with a tongue tip (*see* tongue bath, page 120): moreover, unlike a man, she has two mouths to kiss with, and some women use them beautifully. Eyelashes too can be used for nipple, lip, glans, and skin kisses.

If he hasn't at least kissed her mouth, shoulders, neck, breasts, armpits, fingers, palms, toes, soles, navel, genitals, and earlobes, he hasn't really kissed her: it's no trouble to fill in the gaps for the sake of completeness and makes a touching compliment. And there is no reason why she shouldn't do the same for him.

A good mouth kiss should leave its recipient breathless but not asphyxiated (leave an airway open), and nobody likes their nose squashed into their face. Clean your teeth before making love, and if you are having whisky, garlic, and so on, both of you have it.

pattes d'araignée

Literally "spider's legs"; the French description of tickling erotic massage using the pulps of the fingers with the lightest possible touch, aiming to stimulate not so much the skin as the almost invisible skin hairs: not on the genitals, but all the next most sensitive places – nipples and around, neck, chest, belly, insides of arms and thighs, armpits, hollow of the back, soles and palms, scrotum, space between it and the anus. Use both hands; keep a steady progression of movement going with one, and make surprise attacks with the other.

The whole essence is in the extreme lightness of the touch – more electric than tickling. Feathers (*see* page 113), skin gloves (*see* page 230), or vibrators (*see* pages 262–4) deliver a quite different sensation. If you are agile, don't forget you have toes as well as fingers, and hair in various places, including the eyelashes, to vary the sensation; the real and original French style using the fingertips is difficult to learn but unforgettable by either sex. It's one of the two general skin stimulants (the other is the tongue bath – *see* page 120) that work even on not very skin-conscious males.

pattes d'araignée

*the whole essence is in
the extreme lightness
of the touch*

friction rub

The original meaning of shampoo, which is gentle kneading massage all over. Much more pleasant if you rub each other all over with a condom-compatible massage oil. Sit on something that doesn't matter and rub together or in turns. (Steer well clear of vulnerable body parts like scars and infected skin, and never put firm pressure on organs or on places where the bone is near the skin.) She kneads his muscles, with fingers and a vibrator as well if they like; he concentrates on her breasts, buttocks, loins, and neck. With practice, these sensations are well worth cultivating.

feathers
try soft feathers for exoticism, wiry feathers for arousal

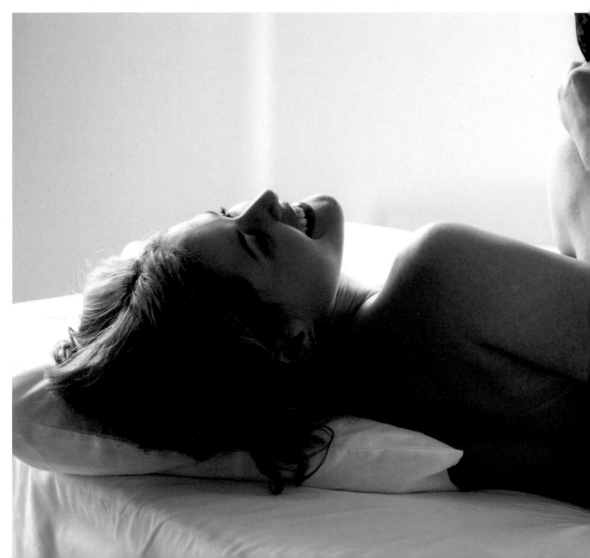

This always ends in genital hand work, then intercourse, followed by a bath together. Semen would be the ideal medium in this context, but sadly it's a case of too little and too late. Bottled lotion, however, offers a practical substitute for this particular fantasy.

feathers

Recommended by some for skin stimulation (of breasts, body surface generally, more than the actual genitals, and palms and soles). Try soft feathers, such as peacock feathers, for exoticism, stiff wiry feathers for arousal, or the feather "mops" sold in sex shops (*see pattes d'araignée*, page 110).

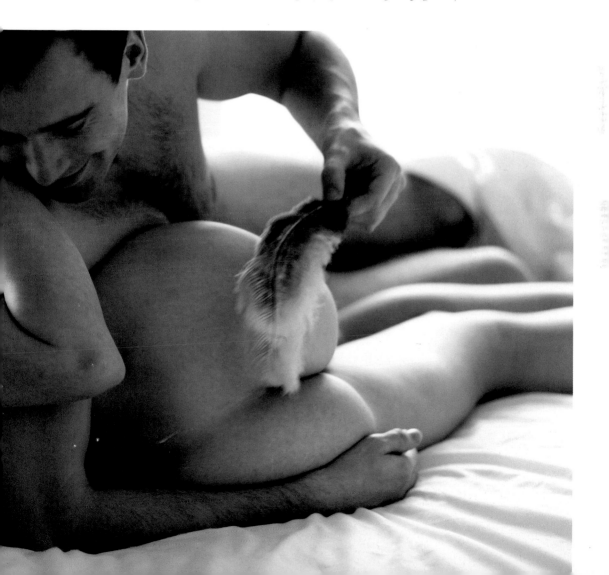

aphrodisiacs

History and urban myth are littered with mentions of "aphrodisiac" foods — these are either symbolic (phallic asparagus and so on), olfactory (fish, tomatoes straight off the plant, which smell sexy), or magical (Brazilian women were reputedly told to pour coffee through their panties and then get their boyfriends to drink it). The *Kama Sutra* recommends spicy foods; Casanova relied on oysters; Aztec king Montezuma claimed it was the fifty cups of hot chocolate he drank a day that kept him capable of serving his harem.

It's an understandable obsession. Desire is so vital and lack of desire so devastating that humankind desperately wants to know the secret of creating and controlling it. Until recently, however, it has been the stuff of dreams; the active ingredients in most reputed aphrodisiacs, including the aforementioned chocolate, are actually so small that they would have little effect, and the ones that work by overstimulation — such as traditional Spanish fly and its modern counterpart, amyl nitrate — can be life-threatening.

In this respect, we have a lot to thank current pharmacology for. Testosterone for both, dopamine for her, an upcoming nasal spray that activates brain receptors; no point in being more specific — the landscape will have changed even before this book goes to press. Particularly intriguing is the idea of the antidepressant that caused research subjects to climax uncontrollably whenever they yawned, though it doesn't sound altogether practical if one gets tired or bored on a regular basis.

Science is only just discovering that emotion can also be an aphrodisiac. While festering anger and real fear kill desire, mild versions of each can have the opposite effect. Hence couples who leap into bed after a fight, hence the effect of edgy sex where uncertainty breeds passion, and "safe" anxiety breeds arousal. Grief, surprisingly, has an effect too; if you find yourselves making love after a recent bereavement, you are neither heartless nor unusual but affirming life in the most fundamental of ways.

In the end, for regular use, most lovers will simply take Euripides' advice and have just a little wine for lubrication and relaxation, along with their food of choice. Because here's the real secret: aphrodisiacs work largely because you think they will. If caviar, champagne, and strawberries create the right mood for you, they will work; if a hamburger and fries are set in the context of "tonight's the night," they will work just as well. No aphrodisiac, it should be added, is a lifesaver or comes up to the combined effect of "the time and the place and the loved one together."

fantasy

The reality is that most of us fantasize – 90 percent of women and almost 100 percent of men. Psychologists would call it a bridge between forbidden urges and the socialized and civilized part of us – the child gets to play, to love, to rebel, to hurt, and to be hurt, but safely and while staying "good." Physiologists would say that it pump-primes: as the brain dreams, the body responds – the tendency to fantasize may be linked with testosterone, which would probably explain the gender difference. But don't take that difference too seriously – some men, particularly under stress, hardly fantasize at all, while in some women, fantasy on its own can trigger orgasm.

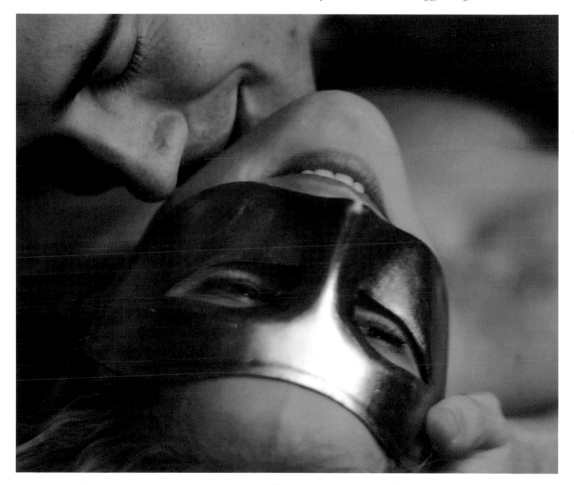

fantasy
as the brain dreams, the body responds

Let's demolish some myths here and now; fantasy isn't the refuge of the undersexed or those who aren't getting it – the more arousable and experienced we are, the more we are likely to fantasize. We may sometimes get spooked, yet such dreams are nothing to be scared of and almost always we fantasize not as a step to doing something in real life but because we never will. (Nighttime dreams, which feel infinitely more alarming because they feel completely outside of our control, are equally safe.) What we do want is to direct our own movie, with ourselves in the starring role – being worshipped, being taken, having sex with someone unavailable, doing things that are forbidden, and all of these in the middle of the high street, at the top of the Empire State Building, with the entire starting lineup of our home team or with all the cheerleaders. We know it will never happen – that would be the point, and also the reassurance.

If the idea appeals but you have difficulty even beginning, it may be that you feel you need to be "creative." Relax – this is not an Oscar winner you are directing, and in any case, all fantasy has its starting point in real life; turn to a strong personal memory (or a favorite piece of erotica), rerun, replay – and then adapt. She is more likely to make a story of it. He is more likely to have single scenes, often with different partners. The key is letting the film roll, no hesitation. This is where you get to be in complete control.

As for telling each other, that's not compulsory – though if silence is guilt-based, it's a good idea to at least tell a therapist. Equally, a partner's fantasy that seriously disturbs is a subject for discussion and adjustment; no one should pressure the other to accept what they hate. Uninhibited partners will tell each other about their fantasies (try free-associating just before orgasm if you are shy). Really communicating partners look for them and put them on the menu unannounced – there is no more complete communication. If the thing itself doesn't turn you on equally, the response will. So say one provocative sentence each in turn, to build the story. Set each other homework, to produce an "essay" as foreplay for next time. Ask your partner to tell (or give) you the thing he or she would most like to see you wearing when you come together for lovemaking and then, next time, wear it. After a few big orgasms together, all but the oddest fantasies get to be shared.

It's tempting to think that the best next step is action. But be careful of crossing the bridge from fantasy to reality; the whole point of fantasy is that what you dream about is sometimes what you are rightly wary of doing. In particular, the cold light of day can make "additional players" a threat; if your fantasy is of a threesome, better to close your eyes and pretend that your partner's hands belong to someone else – this is a far safer option than recruiting crowd scenes (*see* foursomes and moresomes, pages 268–9).

Role-play is a different matter, more acceptable because entirely under your control. In the privacy of one's own room – with or without the addition of a few strategic props – play the master, the mistress, the handsome doctor, or the winsome country maid. He can be the Turkish sultan, whose chosen concubine enters the bedchamber naked and in darkness dives under the covers at the foot of the bed, wriggling her way up alongside him to await his pleasure. She can equally well be Gulbeyaz – the sultan's wife in Byron's *Don Juan* – receiving a favored stud. Take it in turns.

breathing

Not just a mystic ritual – though the *Kama Sutra* focuses on it – but a way of connecting before sex. Standing, sitting, or lying, use belly-to-belly breathing. Keep going until you are in sync, then slow down together, breath by breath, until deep and steady. (If breath is unpleasant, cut back on spicy food and cigarettes; if it still causes a flinch, book a dental appointment.)

To move to arousal, breathe in and up as if through the top of the head; then let the breath go with an audible sound, pelvis rocking slightly forwards, pelvic floor muscles pulling up (*see pompoir*, page 188). Done before lovemaking, this Tantric "fire breath" quickly builds sexual energy; done during the act, it helps you move together.

Use breathing, too, in order to pace orgasm. He can breathe through the nose and into his belly, slowly and steadily, to fool his body into holding back; once ready to push towards climax, he should then shift to short, sharp mouth breathing. Her added trick, when finding it hard to come, is to do whatever she is not doing – either holding her breath rather than letting it go or vice versa.

For some, arousal is linked not to breathing but actively to not breathing; block access to oxygen and adrenaline naturally kicks in to boost sensation. The Inuit knew this long ago; the French Foreign Legionnaires brought it back to Europe from their wars in Indo-China. You may already stop breathing spontaneously at the moment of climax; to replicate this deliberately, simply hold your breath as you hit the point of no return (*see* plateau phase, page 183). But even if asked, don't block a partner's airway; the asphyxiation in the 1970s erotic film classic *Ai no Corrida* may look sensuous, but he dies in the end. So let's not go into detail about how; get the same sensation safely by intercourse head-down (*see* inversion, page 161).

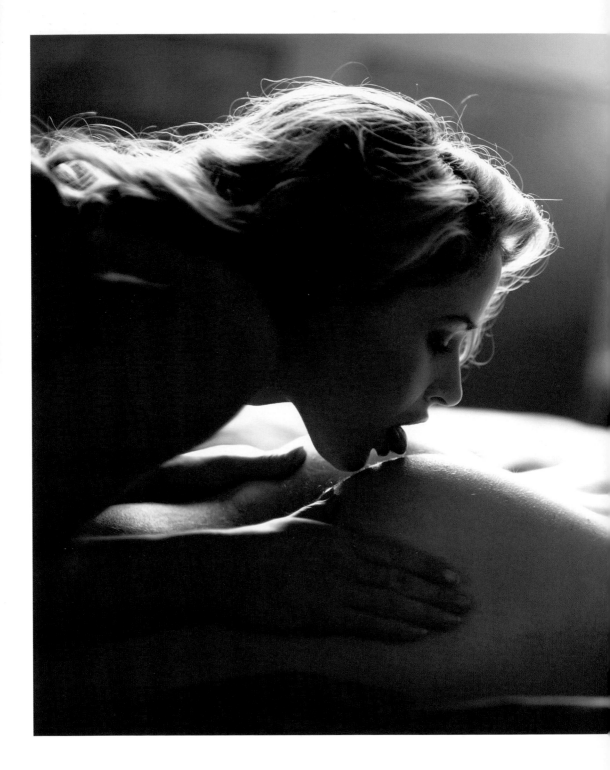

tongue bath
going systematically over
every square inch of a
partner with long, slow,
broad tongue strokes

blowing
can drive some
people out of
their mind

tongue bath

Going systematically over every square inch of a partner, tied if they like, with long, slow, broad tongue strokes – keep a glass of water handy to moisten your mouth, or bite your tongue gently to keep saliva flowing. Start behind, turn them, and cover the front surface after, so as to be in position to go on to coition or hand and mouth work. If the woman gives this, she does it with the man free or staked out, then covers the whole available surface equally systematically with slow strokes of her open vulva followed by leisurely stimulation or riding astride – the whole package reputedly making up the woman's ploy in traditional Croatian intercourse. Mini versions cover particular areas in the same way.

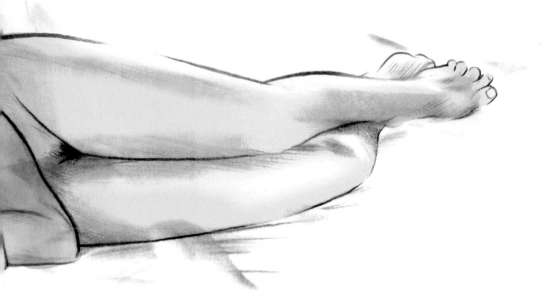

blowing

Not the slang sense (*see* mouth work, pages 136–41), but quite simply making a current of air on the (preferably pre-wetted) skin of any part of the body, either from the lips or from a hair dryer on a cool setting. The best way to moisten an erogenous area is with the tongue, though one could simply begin as a partner emerges from shower or bath; for more extensive operations, use lotion or water sprayed from the sort of fine mister used for house plants. Alternatively, most sex shops supply variations on tingling rubs and sprays.

Air on a wet sensitive surface produces a sensation that can drive some people of either sex out of their mind – experiment on a small scale, using your natural equipment (saliva and breath). In the case of earlobes, breathe in, not out, or you will deafen your partner. Elsewhere, use steady, continuous exhalation with the lips about an inch from the skin. The natural sequel to a tongue bath (*see* opposite). For a bigger operation, use the hair dryer – the result is far wilder than the conventional routine with feathers, except for palms and soles – try mixing the two by hitching a couple of feathers to the dryer nozzle on threads (*see* feathers, page 113). Some words of warning: never use a strong air source (*see* inflators, page 250, and, hazards, pages 260–1), and never blow into the vagina or any other body orifice (except the mouth).

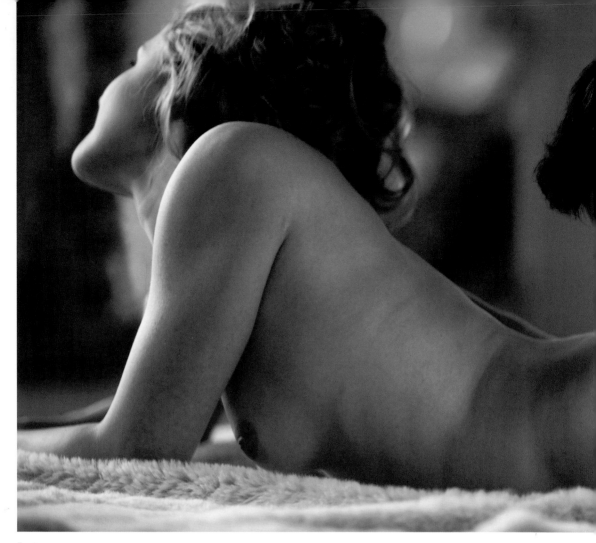

bites

Hindu eroticians classified these at huge length. Gentle nibbling (of the penis, breasts, skin, fingers, ears, labia, clitoris, armpit hair) is part of the general excitatory repertoire. Hard bites at the moment of orgasm excite some people, but for most, like other over-painful stimuli, they are a turnoff. Some people tend to bite more than others; remember that often your partner will do to you what they really want done to them – being aware of this is the great secret of communicating sex.

Love bruises, on the neck and elsewhere, which some lovers find act like a constant playback, setting off more lovemaking every time they are seen, aren't made by biting but by strong, continuous suction kisses; practice on your palm. Check before starting that it's acceptable to leave a mark – if not, make the suction slight. If it goes too far, the application of

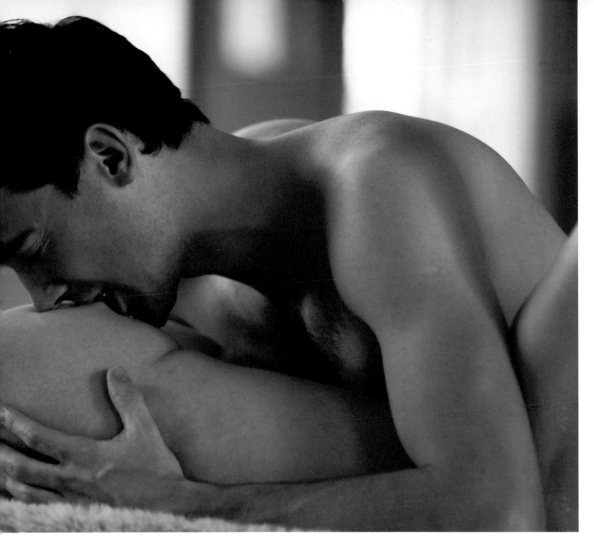

bites
gentle nibbling, hard bites, love bruises

an ice cube will ease out the damage, then use arnica and cover with makeup. Sharper nips to the skin aren't as a rule erotic.

Be careful of biting genitals at all, or any part of the body at or near orgasm; the jaws may go into spasm and you can clamp down really hard – in fact, don't ever have an orgasm with a breast, penis, clitoris, or finger in your mouth. The need to bite can be taken out on something neutral like cloth or hair, and should always be if there is any risk of unsafe sex. This seems to be a case where the mammalian program of reflexes is over-tough for human enjoyment.

l'onanisme

However much sex you have, you will probably still want simple, own-hand masturbation – not only during periods of separation but simply when you feel like another orgasm, or feel like having a different experience of being in control of your own body. (She may also use it to ease period pain or bring an end to menstruation.)

Originally the subject of uninhibited celebration – the ancient Egyptians thought that their entire world had been created from the god Atum's masturbatory ejaculation – self-pleasuring soon began to get bad press. The critical comments began when humankind realized that semen was linked

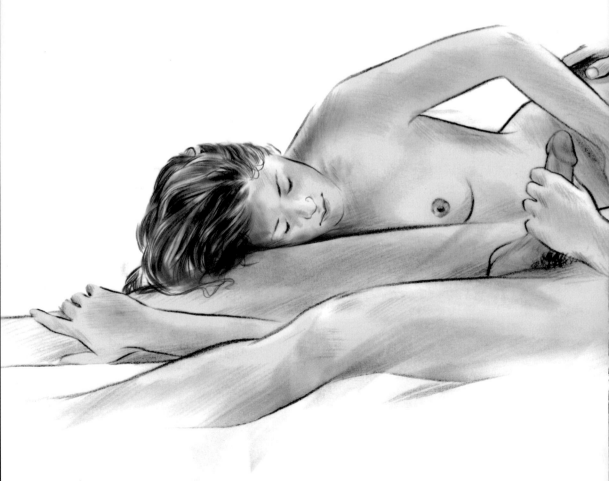

with conception and the religious texts started claiming that "spilling seed" was wasteful; then eighteenth-century Swiss physician Samuel-Auguste Tissot linked masturbation with blurred vision and fueled an enduring – and utterly erroneous – myth. Today, the hang-ups are different, but still as strong, so let's be clear: if one masturbates it doesn't mean one has a bad sex life and if one's partner masturbates it doesn't mean that he (or she) isn't satisfied. Solo masturbation is different from couple sex, but not inferior, in the same way as oral sex is different from intercourse; we can – perhaps even should – indulge in and enjoy both.

l'onanisme
climaxing solo in front of a partner is one of the biggest gifts you can give

Whether alone or together, don't settle into habit. One's own preferred way will be quicker and easier, but can make for less flexibility around routes to orgasm – variety will keep all options open. So change, as a matter of habit. Shift position, grind into a pillow, use a dildo in whatever orifice, play in the bath, experiment with a vibrator. All these are instructions to him and to her. The Internet has a thousand more suggestions.

Loving couples don't just accept each other's masturbatory patterns, but welcome them as a way to learn; climaxing solo in front of a partner is one of the biggest gifts you can give. He needs to observe closely; pioneering sex researchers Masters and Johnson report never having seen two women do it exactly the same way. She needs to accept that his masturbatory force is focus, not aggression; if she is aroused by it rather than wary of it, that will move everything to a higher plane.

Some women feel left out or rejected if they find their partner masturbating; if you feel vibrations when he thinks you are asleep and want to get in on the act, finish him yourself at full speed, or better, start slow, then stop, tie him, and make him watch you masturbate yourself, slowly and with style, before you put him out of his misery. The unexpected sight of a woman giving herself an orgasm when he can't move is unbearably exciting for most men. Make sure he can't get loose. Watching each other take the last orgasm separately but together makes a great end to any session.

fighting

The occasional arguments that all lovers experience would have nothing to do with sex if some couples weren't directly excited by them, often without knowing it – that real anger has erotic effects is a matter of true folklore. But let's be clear. Neither she nor he should ever put up with real violence or anything that doesn't stop when you say stop – this kind of behavior will continue or more usually escalate, however much the aggressor apologizes (*see* resources, pages 276–91). Real, spiteful violence from a partner is a common cause of death or injury. Don't put up with it, and don't give any second chances – leave and/or go to the police. Sadistic bullies are incurable by love.

Back to the main route. As we have several times remarked, our image of love is uptight about the elements of forcefulness that exist in normal sexuality – which makes us prone to mix erotic energy with real spite or real anger, and confuse two quite distinct things. To need some degree of energy in sex, rather than the glutinous, unphysical kind of love that the tradition propagates, is statistically pretty normal. But the way to meet this need isn't to use fights to fuel it, but rather to learn the purposive uses of play. True, the over-gentle spouse is likely to be blocked about aggression, and nonplussed by the demand "Now take me." He (or she) has probably been taught not to treat a partner like that – if he is excessively over-gentle, in fact, he may be sitting on a strong need to do so. But if these things can once be talked about, you can help him (or her) learn the uses of sexual play without the need to mix it up with real day-to-day angers and frustrations that can get out of hand. If he is over-gentle, don't needle him, teach him.

With a normally energetic partner, don't be ashamed if you really argue (most people do), but don't treat it as a kick, or a way of turning on a partner's sexual arousal. Use play. Cultivate pillow talk to unblock fantasies – ask each other just short of orgasm: "What would you like to do to me, like me to do to you, now?" – "now" meaning at the fantasy level (*see* bird-song at morning, pages 194–5). As nearly always with human beings, symbolisms are generally bigger kicks than over-literal enactments.

Separately, some couples get a lot of fun out of extended struggles, pre-meditated or impromptu – "love wrestling" in the old tradition. (It's maybe why same-sex wrestling – often with the addition of mud – is seen as a turn-on nowadays, and also why Sumo wrestlers are significant sex symbols in their own country.) Enthusiasts go in for elaborate handicaps: time limits, no biting or scratching, and so on. Most people find fairly robust but reasonable tussling quite enough, others play elaborate finding-fault-and-spanking games (don't play these over real faults). Women (and men) who enjoy an extra sensation of helplessness differ whether they feel this more held down or tied up: either sex can take out quite a lot of the energy component in the actual process of working for orgasm. Once understood, none of this range of needs is scary, and can be stopped spilling out of sex into cruelty, or the normal resentments felt by any two people who live together. Actually, it tends to discharge these.

Nothing we have said excludes the tenderness of sex. If you haven't learned that sexual energy can be tender and tenderness forceful, you haven't begun to play as real lovers. If you do have a real fight, make sure to end it in bed. At least it's the best way to finish.

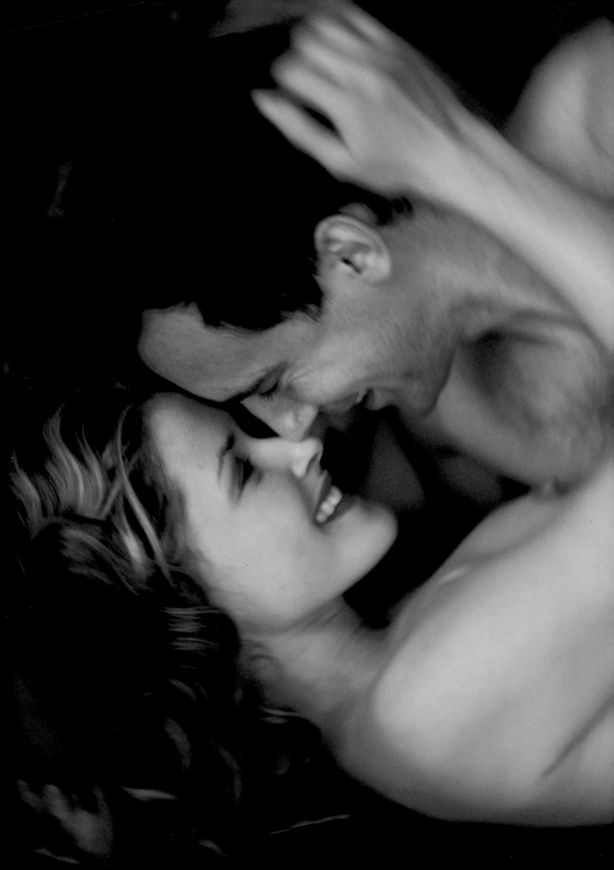

main
courses

postures

Endless time has been spent throughout history, chiefly by non-playing coaches, in describing and giving fancy names to upwards of six hundred of these – collecting them is obviously a human classificatory hobby. Most of the non-extreme postures come naturally, and few of the extreme ones merit more than a single visit out of curiosity. The only part we regret is the loss of the fancy names, Arabic, Sanskrit, or Chinese, that they have been given across cultures and down the centuries.

Most people now know the obvious ones and have learned which make for quick and slow orgasm and how to use them in series. A few people, either for symbolic or anatomical reasons, can only achieve an orgasm in one or two of them.

Inspection will indicate which of these fit special situations, such as pregnancy, disability, height differences, and so on. Only trial will indicate which work best, or at all, orgasm-wise. Couples frequently start by trying the whole lot, but nearly inevitably end up with one or two, going back to the book for special occasions.

Some of the really wild fantasies in Oriental manuscripts do have a point – the woman astride in Mughal pictures who is balancing lighted lamps on her hands, head, and shoulders or shooting at a target with a bow is only showing that she can bring the man off with her vaginal muscles alone while keeping the rest of her still (*see pompoir*, page 188). Others are mystical or merely gymnastic. All the poses we show are practicable (and have been tried for fit, if not to orgasm) and more or less rewarding according to inclination. What we do suggest is that for any new trick you arrange a practice session in anticipation. The time to learn new figures isn't on the ice rink or

postures
even the most accomplished musician has to practice, though in love, once learned is never forgotten

the dance floor. The most common reason that an elaboration you both wanted — whether it's a fancy posture or some dodge such as bondage, which needs to be quickly and efficiently set up — disappoints is the attempt to use it in actual, excited lovemaking "from cold," so that you mess about, lose the thread, and wish you hadn't bothered with it or blame whoever suggested it. The usual and regrettable outcome is never to try again.

Not that rehearsal need be cold-blooded or taken out of actual love-making. Anticipation being good in itself, you first fantasize about it, sit down together, plan, and rehearse. Then fit the actual trial-for-size into the waiting periods between bouts — when you are both excited enough not to feel silly, but not ready to go completely: try it while waiting for the next erection. Remember, even the most accomplished musician has to practice, though in love, once learned is never forgotten. If it works the first time, you should get the erection — in that case, go where it takes you. This means

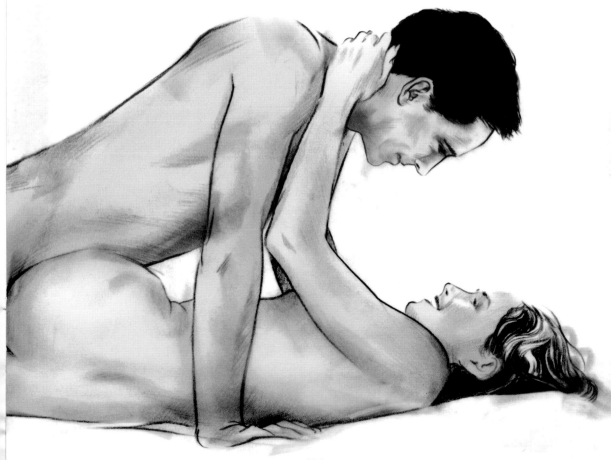

131

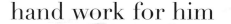

hand work for him

A woman who has the divine gift of lechery and loves her partner will masturbate him well, and a woman who knows how to masturbate a man – subtly, unhurriedly, and mercilessly – will almost always make a superlative partner. She needs intuitive empathy and real enjoyment of a penis, holding it in just the right place, with just the right amount of pressure and movement, timing her action in bursts to coincide with his feeling – stopping or slowing to keep him in suspense, speeding up to control his climax. Some men can't stand really proficient masturbation to climax unless securely tied (*see* rope work, pages 256–7) and virtually none can hold still for slow masturbation (*see* slow masturbation for him, pages 269–71).

The variation can be endless, even if she doesn't have the choice of foreskin back, foreskin not back, which again yield two quite distinct nuances. If he isn't circumcised, she will probably need to avoid rubbing the glans itself, except in pursuit of very special effects. Her best grip is just below the groove, with the skin back as far as it will go, and using two hands – one holding the penis steady, or fondling the scrotum, the other making a thumb-and-first-finger ring, or a whole-hand grip. She should vary this

hand work for him

*a woman who knows how to masturbate a man –
subtly, unhurriedly, and mercilessly – will almost
always make a superlative partner*

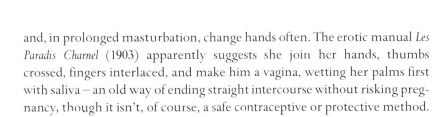

and, in prolonged masturbation, change hands often. The erotic manual *Les Paradis Charnel* (1903) apparently suggests she join her hands, thumbs crossed, fingers interlaced, and make him a vagina, wetting her palms first with saliva – an old way of ending straight intercourse without risking pregnancy, though it isn't, of course, a safe contraceptive or protective method.

For a full orgasm, she sits comfortably on his chest or kneels astride him. During every extended sexual session, one orgasm – usually the second or third if he is lasting for that long – is well worth giving in this particular way: the French professionals who used no other method didn't only stay in business through fear of infection. It's well worth devoting time and effort to perfecting this technique – it fully expresses love, and can be domesticated in any bedroom.

Rolling the penis like pastry between the palms of two hands is another technique, best used for producing an erection rather than going for orgasm. For some occasions she can try to copy his own favorite method of self-masturbation. When she uses her own rhythm it can have a different and sometimes more startling effect.

mouth work for her

In the first half of the twentieth century, genital kisses, or rather the taboos on them, were a king pretext for divorce on grounds of perversity, cruelty, and so on. We have come some way since then – now there are textbooks on them, and they figure in films. Personal likes and dislikes apart, most people now know that, given safety constraints (*see* safe sex, pages 96–8), they are one of the best things in sexual intimacy. Who goes first is clearly a matter of preference, but one can give the woman dozens of purely preliminary orgasms in this way, as many as she can take, and she will still want to go on from there, so the man had better save himself for later.

mouth work for her
give the woman dozens of pre-
liminary orgasms and she will
still want to go on from there

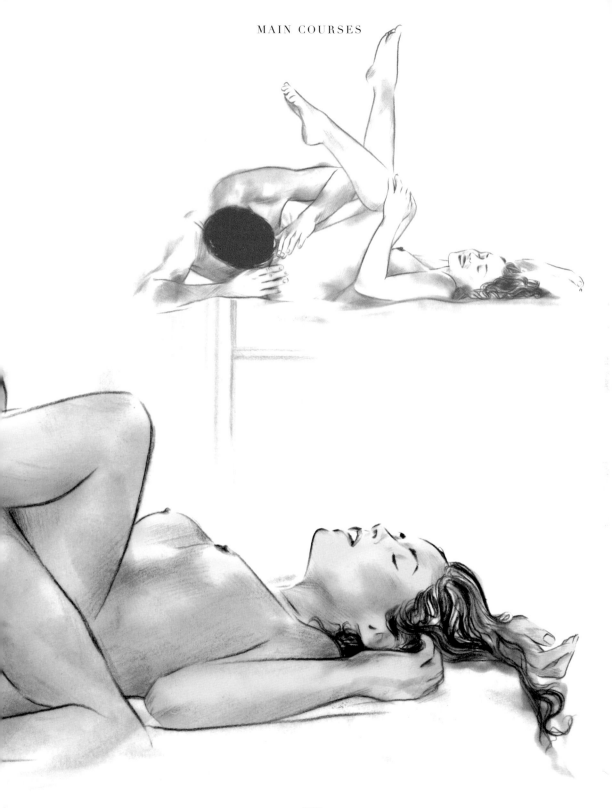

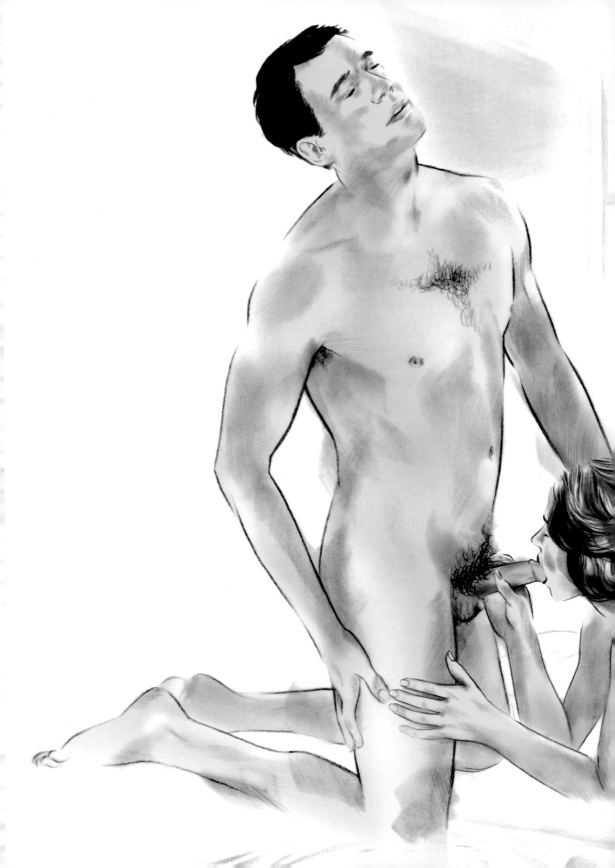

hates it but because she can't help herself. A large penis will also stretch the mouth quite a lot, so be considerate." In this respect, pulling her head towards him without permission is one of the few almost unforgivable bedroom sins. He should always be sure to let her stay in control of the pace and depth of the kiss.

There are a minority of men who are unable to experience even the briefest of genital kisses before uncontrollably ejaculating – these should reserve it until they require a new erection, when it is a uniquely effective way of raising the dead.

mouth work for him
one of the most moving gestures in the whole sexual experience

clitoral pleasure

Unless you have been trapped in the jungle for the past fifty years, you are probably aware of what women have always known, experts have often denied, and sex researcher Shere Hite clearly substantiated in the mid-twentieth century: it's clitoral stimulation that delivers most female orgasms. For this reason, we devote a few paragraphs here to the topic.

Let's start with the question of validity. Those (usually male) sexologists who suggest that a vaginal orgasm is a signal of a more mature sexuality are ignoring two things. First, the biology of the situation, which suggests that as penis and clitoris are equivalent – which we now know they are – it's the clitoris one should be addressing if one wants to get the same brisk response from a woman as from a man. Second, female experience, which consistently endorses the fact that most women climax easily, quickly, and without stress from clitoral stimulation, whereas intercourse typically demands effort, concentration, and either a carefully chosen range of positions or – here we come back to square one – a clitorally targeted helping hand.

Given all this, the dedicated male player who longs to know what to do with a clitoris can do worse than refer back to his own, larger version. Movements with finger or tongue up and down the shaft, quick flicks across the tip, gentle sucking of the glans, highly targeted pressure on the "frenulum equivalent" where the hood retracts; these will all work as well for her as for him. He doesn't need to be clever, just follow his own instincts. One caveat only; scale down for size. Where he may like rough, she will seldom want anything but gentle and lubricated, which is why tongue work is often her medium of choice.

Does intercourse ever achieve the same effect? Of course it does – the symbolism alone makes it central to the whole performance. Many women whose physiology permits get supreme climaxes this way, and those penetration positions that stretch or nudge the clitoris (see CAT, page 193) are highly functional. But to solve this particular conundrum, most couples combine, choosing positions that allow hand or vibrator access – her on top or rear entry for preference (see upper hands, page 158, X position, page 165, rear entry, pages 169–72, and bridge, pages 191–2).

Does intercourse alone work? Not necessarily, not always – and not if you slide a "should" or a "must" in there with it. Saying that a woman "should" climax with penetration is equivalent to saying that a man "should" climax through having his testicles pulled. Some do, some don't, and in any case each to their own. Defining the way to orgasm for either sex is, in our opinion, a red herring.

soixante-neuf

Both of you delivering mouth work to each other at the same time is fine but has some drawbacks. It needs attention and care to give your partner your best, and consequently you can't go berserk over it, as you can over mutual intercourse: impending orgasm, especially in the woman, just isn't compatible with careful technique, and the man can even be bitten. Another slight but, for some men, real defect is that in *soixante-neuf* the woman is the wrong way round for tongue work on the most sensitive surface of the glans (this explains the acrobatics in some Indian temple statues, which aim to get both mutuality and a better approach for the woman). Mutual genital kisses are wonderful, but if you are going to orgasm, it's usually better to take turns.

For some couples, the simultaneous, sixty-nine-type kiss really does represent the ultimate in sensation. Since loss of control will be complete, he should check first that she can handle his ejaculating into her mouth. The woman-on-top position in most books is all right, especially if she combines mouth work with hand work, but it gives the man a stiff neck. Especially good is the no-cushions position – head to tail on their sides, each with the under thigh drawn up as a cushion for the partner's head. The man can open her widely by slipping his arm in the crook of her upper knee.

The mutual kiss can be long or short; the short is just in passing – the long can last minutes or hours according to taste and speed. Both fit nicely between rounds of intercourse, as well as acting as hors d'oeuvres or alternatively a corpse reviver.

If, on the other hand, they are going alternately, let him start, preferably in this same no-cushions position, while she does very little. Then it can be her turn; or they can go on to intercourse, putting off fellatio until he has had one orgasm and a rest and is due for his next erection. In this way she can abandon herself, and watch her technique when she sucks him.

birth control

The discovery that more than any other made carefree sex possible was hormonal contraception. Before that, it was down to plugging her vagina with crocodile dung or covering his penis with a length of animal intestine – and even then anxiety made impossible the kind of extended sexual play that's now available to everyone. As the saying went, couples sowed their wild oats on Saturday night and on Sunday prayed for crop failure. Women who have experienced the security of modern methods and discovered the play function of sex are not going to return willingly to the old insecurity. Neither are their partners.

The (justifiable) price of such freedom, however, is that for any methods apart from condoms, we now need expert guidance for prescription and usage. What follows, consequently, is not in-depth coverage – that should come from a health professional as part of a consultation (*see* resources, pages 276–9) – but the Cook's Tour for orientation purposes.

The pill is still the overall contraceptive of choice, despite its reliance on a good memory. Hormonal injections, implants, patches – and all variations and combinations thereof – work in roughly the same way and with the same effect, but don't need to be remembered daily. Injections and implants are more permanent and so she needs to know that she won't react badly to the hormones before going that route. Emergency contraception can be taken up to seventy-two hours (the pill) or five days (an IUD) after sex, useful at times of contraceptive disaster; an option used not, as the myths suggest, by irresponsible teens but in reality by forty-somethings whose lives are so rushed that they forget the pill or split the condom.

Intrauterine devices (IUDs) placed at the neck of the womb allow for spontaneity; the new hormonal versions offer even greater reliability. All these methods are reversible given time; the question is whether she wants to ingest hormones – which do guard against some diseases, even if they may make others more likely. If she suffers side effects, she should consult her health professional; a different prescription is often the answer.

Diaphragms and caps offer less efficacy, but also fewer hormones. Some women find that capping themselves before sex is off-putting; some get resistance from partners (though if it's the only method she can use, don't make a song and dance about it; that won't change anything and will make her apprehensive). Either diaphragm or cap can also, handily, hold back menstrual blood if you want intercourse during her period.

The condom, male and female, has the overwhelming selling point of being the only method that offers true safe-sex protection. Hence ignore its reputation as being the "starter" contraceptive and take full advantage; in any but established (and tested) relationships, you are best to use them even if already using hormonal methods. The manipulation involved in letting the woman put a condom on her man excites some people – for a real party trick she can position it with finger and thumb, then roll it down with her tongue. Some makes of knobbed or otherwise-decorated male condoms sold to vary vaginal sensation are unreliable; check the packet for quality-tested logos. They can also slow down some over-quick ejaculators. For guidelines on use, *see* safe sex, pages 96–8.

Vasectomy and sterilization are the once-and-for-all contraceptive methods of choice. The male version blocks the tubes down which the sperm travel from the testes, the female version blocks the tubes through which the sperm travel to meet the egg. His operation is done under local anesthetic, hers is a much more major procedure; with both there is a slight time delay before real protection kicks in and neither guarantees any safety when it comes to infections. Plus, you can't easily change your mind, so regard both options as irreversible, and if you are hesitating about the decision, don't do it. However, it's now possible to store sperm or eggs for use at a later date should circumstances change.

If religious beliefs dictate the rhythm method (*coitus reservatus* or "Vatican roulette"), use it carefully and accurately for any serious chance of reliability. The same, only more so, applies to withdrawal (*coitus interruptus*); by the time he is ready to climax fully, he will already have oozed more than enough sperm to make her pregnant a few thousand times over. Regard with equal terror other mythical measures: sex during her period, douching, sneezing, urinating afterwards, and doing it standing up.

If she is unhappily pregnant, seek medical advice immediately; whether or not there is a decision to be made, it's best to have expert support early on. In many countries, abortion is now medically a less traumatic procedure than it was, but that doesn't necessarily make it less emotionally traumatic; get support both before and after in order to preempt any emotional kickbacks. That doesn't just mean for her; he may be grieving too.

In most situations there is no reason not to use contraception, so if you aren't, it's likely to be because of what you are feeling rather than what you are doing. This is not a scolding, but an invitation to consider that if one or both of you keep making a "mistake," it's not really a mistake. You want to have a baby – for someone to love, for someone to love you, to keep up with your friends, to keep hold of your partner. There is nothing bad about any of these motives, but being aware of them will mean it's much more likely that you will make the life choices you really want to make.

birth control
the manipulation involved in
letting the woman put a condom
on her man excites some people

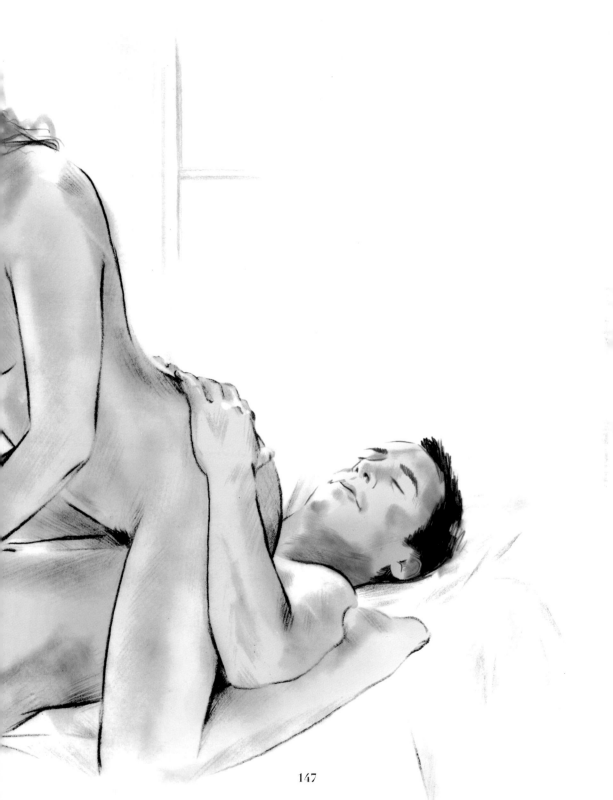

penetration

Love, closeness, abandoning oneself to one's partner, surrendering (for him), embracing (for her). Reaction to penetration is a summary of who you are individually and in relation to each other. Because of all that, it's the most powerful, most unifying sexual act.

And hence, it always needs approaching with respect on both sides and only when there is full arousal on hers. A courteous lover will pause as he enters, to honor the connection; she, in response, can bear down slightly to welcome him in. Go slow and gentle on the first in-stroke to gauge how much she can take; this will vary according to her mood and often the time of the month. Pulling back slightly, then pushing in a fraction deeper, but still slowly, anchors the connection.

There will be occasions when – for lack of time or her need to be taken brusquely – you don't do any of the above, but thrust in fast and furious. Given happy consent, that's fine too. He may feel more, and there is a unique sensation for her around drier entry – a balance between pain and pleasure – which, if she is emotionally relaxed, can be memorable.

Pain on its own is a different issue. For either him or her, discomfort on penetration can indicate infection or structural problems, and for her, pelvic inflammatory disease, hormonal imbalance, or endometriosis. If the trouble occurs suddenly, and after sufficient arousal and lubrication, see a doctor urgently. This doesn't apply to the sort of pain that happens after a

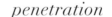

penetration
the most powerful,
most unifying
sexual act

marathon sex session or following a long period of abstinence, when eager-
ness and sheer wear and tear kick in; this is simply your body's way of telling
you to slow down a little.

A stage on from this – vaginismus – means that she closes to the point of
blocking penetration entirely. This is not unusual – some figures suggest
20 percent of women suffer – and is not something to be taken lightly.
Don't attempt treatment by persuasion or seduction, or an exhortation to
"Grit your teeth"; professional support is called for to explore physical and
emotional issues, present and often past (*see* resources, page 276–9).

After the first successful penetration, each withdrawal and reentry –
whether to change position or simply to take time between orgasms – will
give a slightly different set of sensations depending on her varying lubrication or his varying firmness. The early Arabic sex manual *The Perfumed Garden*
lists six distinct ways of penetrating. Long-term partners will probably
develop many more.

choreography

Once joined in whatever position, what remains to be choreographed are
depth, speed, and pattern. And though it may seem as if whoever is on top
sets the agenda, what follows, in fact, will be a subtle communication, a
negotiation between each other's lists of needs and desires. Pulling closer,
pulling away, moving back, hesitating, urging on – all these will be signaled
consciously with touches and murmurs, unconsciously by shifts of breathing and heart rate.

How to decide what is appropriate and when? The myth is that deepest
penetration causes strongest sensation; in reality, it's just one good option
– shallow serves to extend intercourse and in any case should always be
used initially to respect as-yet-not-fully-aroused vaginal tissue. As to speed,
fast may mean a quick ending, while slow can keep both hovering on the
edge of orgasm for hours.

Patterns of varying strokes create varying sensations. The Chinese used
complicated mixtures of deep and shallow, often in magical numbers – five
deep, eight shallow, or such; he could use that basic pattern repeated twice
slowly, then twice at a medium speed, then twice fast, reverting to slow
again. Counting the patterns can help him to control his orgasm, though
the inconsistency may actively interfere with her arousal. If she prefers
unpredictability, however, this will play well for her; he should also pause
occasionally to keep her in anticipation (*see* holding back, page 204).

trigger points

There is much controversy about whether key trigger points – the G-, A-, and U-spot – exist. All that needs to be said is that it's worth exploring. But if she doesn't have them, then it's irrelevant – and anxiety-provoking – to insist that she does or regret that she doesn't, and in any case there are plenty of other ways to please. Here are some signposts.

The G-spot – typically a few inches into her vagina. With fingers, simply reach in and beckon towards her belly button – specially designed vibrators have a curve. For intercourse, you need positions that hit the front vaginal wall: rear entry where she arches her back and widens her legs; front entry where she puts her feet on his chest and arches her pelvis. Go slowly and work around the spot with circular movements; at first she can feel as if she is passing water and may need to relax through it. The result, in some women, may be a spurt of liquid – not urine but female ejaculate.

The A-spot – further into her vagina. Use fingers and vibrator in the same way, but slide in more deeply. For intercourse, positions of choice are rear entry, with her sitting or squatting over him, or front entry with her sitting on the edge of the bed and wrapping her legs around his waist.

The U-spot – the external "spot," situated on her vulva between the clitoris and the vaginal opening. Slow rhythmic pressure is best – she can take charge here and use his penis to bring herself along. Or kneel on top of him (*see* upper hands, page 158) and use her own finger or a vibrator.

missionary position

Name given by amused Polynesians, who preferred squatting intercourse (*see* seated positions, page 179), to the European matrimonial style (*see* pages 156–7). Libel on one of the most rewarding sex positions.

matrimonial
wildly tough or very
tender, slow or quick,
deep or shallow

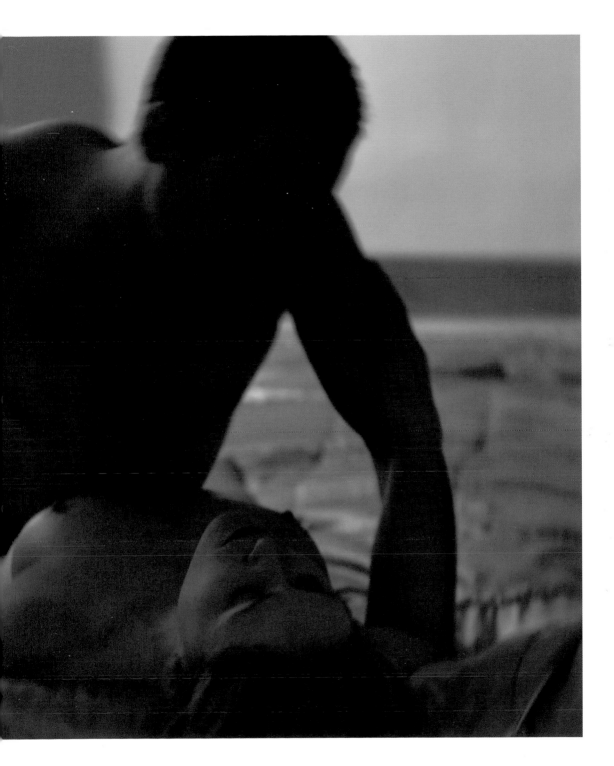

inversion

with orgasm the buildup of pressure in the veins of the face and neck can produce startling sensations

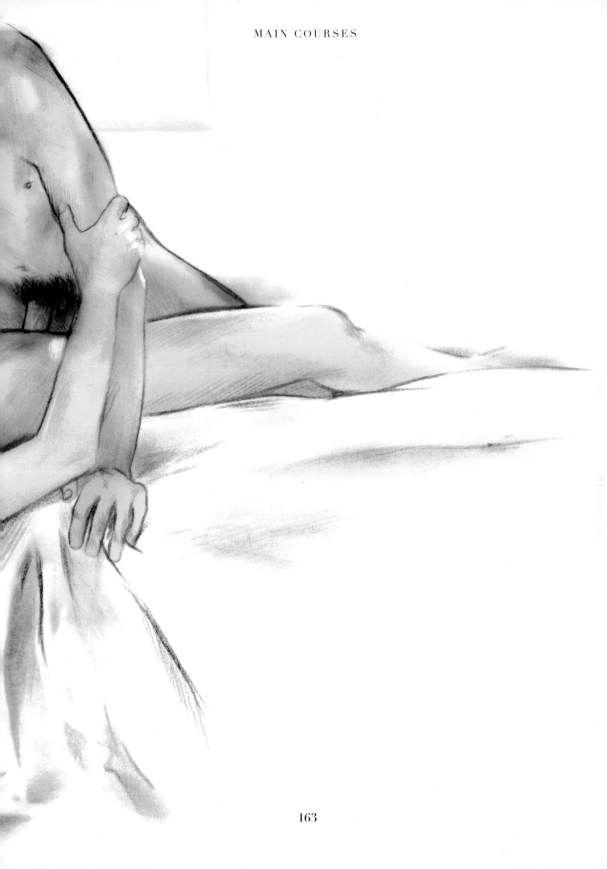

flanquette
extra clitoral pressure
from the man's thigh if he
presses hard with it

X position

A winner for prolonged, slow intercourse. Start with her sitting facing astride him with one or both legs over his, penis fully inserted. She then lies right back – clasping his hands will help – until each partner's head and trunk are horizontal. Slow, coordinated wriggling movements will keep him erect and her close to orgasm for long periods. To switch back to other positions, either of them can sit up without disconnecting. Useful when neither partner can bear weight because of tiredness, illness, or disability. In particular, use as a discreet training position when she is learning to help herself to climax by hand during intercourse and might get embarrassed if he is obviously watching.

X position
a winner for prolonged,
slow intercourse

rear entry
extra depth and buttock stimulation,
hand access to breasts and clitoris,
the sight of her rear view

In the classic version, she kneels on the bed, hands clasped behind her neck, breasts and face down. He kneels behind. She hooks her legs over his and thus pulls him to her – he puts a hand on each of her shoulder blades and presses down. This very deep position is apt to pump her full of air, which escapes later in a disconcerting manner, but is otherwise excellent. He can also hold her breasts or pubis, or, if she likes to be controlled, grasp her wrists behind her. A pile of hard pillows under her middle will help to prevent the position from collapsing if she doesn't like being forcibly held, or she can kneel on the floor with her chest on the bed or a chair seat. The head-down position is best for depth and total apposition – avoid it if it hurts her, if she has a weak back, or if she is pregnant.

Many women like a finger, either his or hers, on the clitoris during inter-course and this is easy to accomplish in all rear positions. It's worth trying in any case, as it totally alters the range of sensation. Grasping the whole pussy in one hand gives a different sensation again and doesn't give the excessive sharpness that comes from strong clitoral stimulation. Alternatively, he can withdraw briefly and give a few clitoral strokes with the glans, guiding it with his hand.

While the deep kneeling position is, or can be, one of the toughest, from behind on your sides is about the gentlest (*à la paresseuse* – the lazy position) and can even be done in sleep – best if she draws her top thigh up a little and sticks her bottom out. This is one position that, for many women, can be managed with very little or even no erection; it can help to cure partial impo-tence or nervousness on the male side by restoring morale. It's also excellent if you want gentle sex for reasons of pregnancy, illness, or disability.

It's well worth experimenting with the full range of rear positions at least as fully as with the face-to-face series, because there almost certainly will be at least one you will use regularly along with the matrimonial, and its variants, and the woman-astride positions.

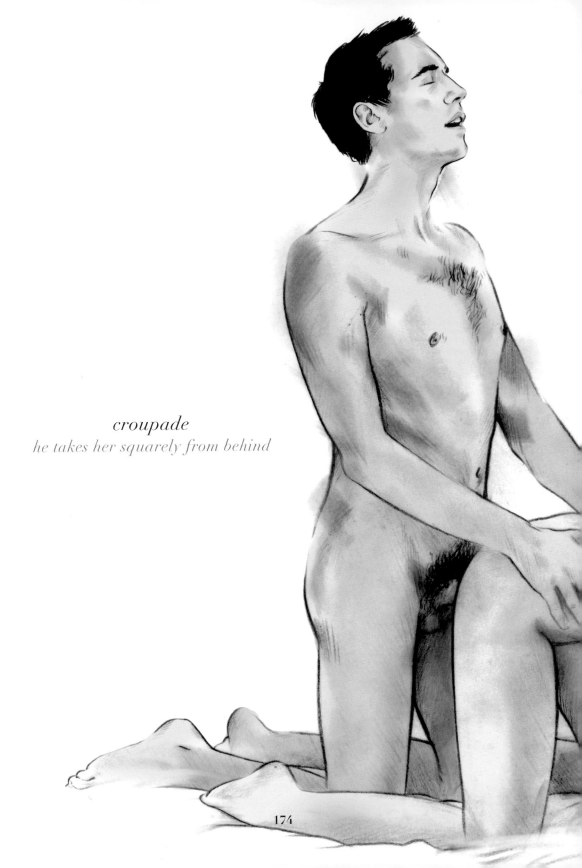

croupade
he takes her squarely from behind

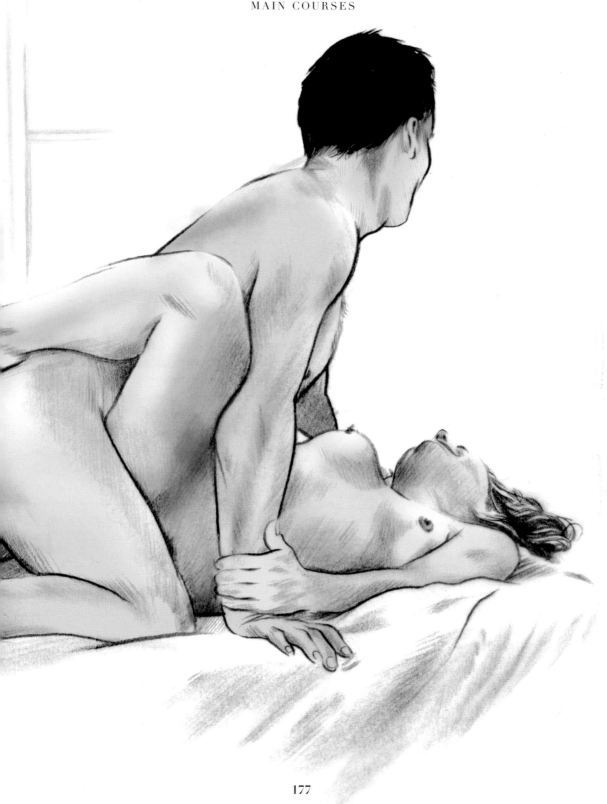

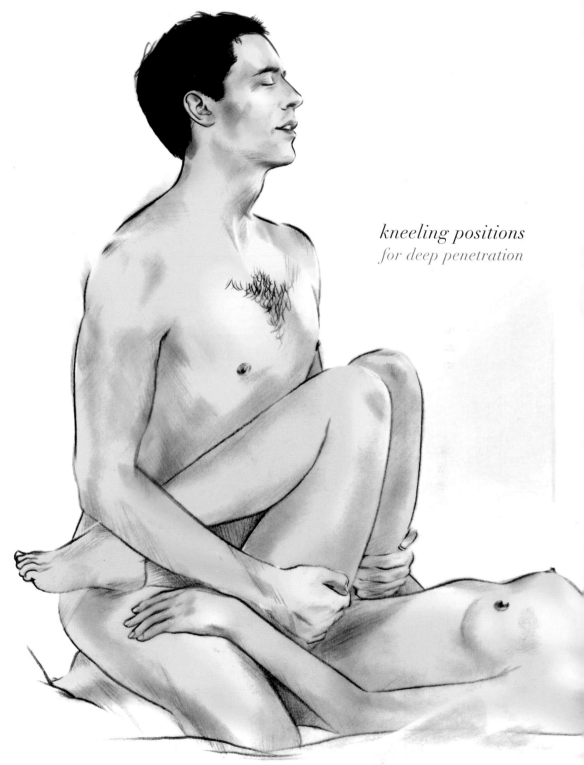

kneeling positions
for deep penetration

kneeling positions

Any intercourse position where one kneels and the other lies back. Hers is largely Hobson's choice, kneeling astride him on top, with her only decision being between facing towards or away. He has more options: her lying flat on the bed, feet on floor; flat on floor with legs up and feet either side of his thighs; feet on his chest; feet around his waist; feet over his shoulders and legs crossed to tighten her vagina. He can also choose whether to kneel up or kneel back on his heels; both demand a soft surface under hard knee bones, and the latter has a limited time span due to cramp – throw down a pillow and aim for five minutes maximum. You can then start to vary where her feet go. Advocates recommend this for when one wants deep penetration and G-spot stimulation (*see* trigger points, page 153).

seated positions

The "pre-missionary" position – the one quite a few cultures favored before they got invaded and forced to do it man-on-top. She sits on the ground with her legs spread, he squats or kneels between them, penetrates, then pulls her towards him; variations include her lying all the way back, her sitting on his lap, or both leaning away with their weight on their hands. Particularly good where one or other partner has a disability that makes prone postures or weight-bearing difficult. The Polynesians preferred this because it makes her orgasm easier – having four hands free helps. The Ghanaian Tallensi preferred it because if the woman wanted out, she could push the man over with a kick – which has a certain appeal. The Chinese reputedly called it "wailing monkey clasping a tree."

If involving furniture – chair, table, car hood – make sure she can lean back against something while she wraps her legs around his waist. Vice versa, he sits on a chair and she straddles; some sex manuals suggest she then puts both ankles on his shoulders, but you would probably need to have circus training for that.

turning positions

Any position where one or both partners switch viewpoint, or begin on top and end up underneath; the *Kama Sutra* warns these are only mastered with practice. Classics are matrimonial (*see* pages 156–7), with him then turning to face her feet, or upper hands (*see* page 158), with her then turning to present her buttocks. The challenge is to keep the connection. If simply reversing superiority, she can put her legs around his waist or intertwine both sets of calves. If one or the other is turning to face in another direction, go for deep penetration followed by careful synchronicity. To be honest, it's usually easier to withdraw, rearrange, and then reinsert.

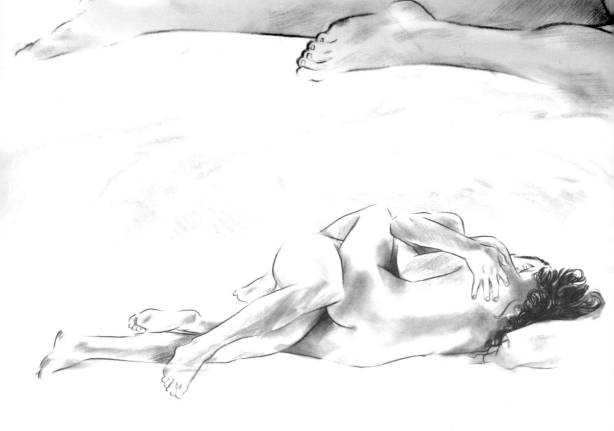

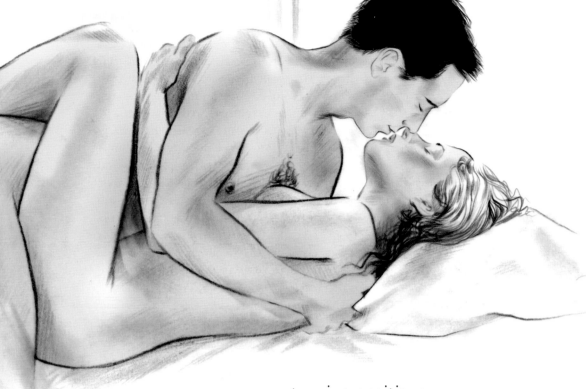

turning positions
the challenge is to keep the connection

Viennese oyster

A woman who can cross her feet behind her head, lying on her back, of course. When she has done so, he holds her tightly around each instep with his full hand and squeezes, lying on her full-length. Don't try to put an unsupple partner into this position – it can't be achieved by brute force. You can get a very similar sensation – unique rocking pelvic movement – with less expertise if she crosses her ankles on her tummy, knees to shoulders, and he lies on her crossed ankles with his full weight. Why "Viennese" we don't know. Tolerable for short periods only and expect only shallow penetration. Worth trying, nevertheless.

sex for pregnancy

Those who know report that sex in the context of baby-making is a very different experience. Realizing that what you are doing aims to create a human life can focus the mind and add an extra dimension of gravitas to the situation, but doesn't mean that the passion should be sidelined.

Which is why it's best to avoid getting hooked on the "how." Yes, it makes sense not to defy gravity by putting her on top or standing, and not to do something obviously stupid like douching. But there is no actual research about which positions work best, while the old wives' tale about the pillow under the buttocks has been actively disproved. All that's certain is that deep positions help – but which is the deepest for any one couple depends how their bits fit, and after that it's a matter for experimentation.

So forget the mechanics. Get health checks for both, get as fit as possible, lose the cigarettes and the alcohol. Then relax. Ninety out of every hundred couples trying to get pregnant do so within two years (for those who don't, *see* resources, pages 276–9, for help), and enjoyable lovemaking will shorten that period more than stressed, obsessive copulation where he feels like a sperm bank and she like a brood mare. If ever there is an argument for remembering the joy of sex, it's here.

Once pregnant, the temptation may be to back off lovemaking – he for fear of damaging her or the baby, she because she feels too nauseous to do anything but curl up and whimper. The second will resolve itself. The first – given a medical all clear – can be ignored; all kinds of orgasm are a good idea, bringing extra blood and hence nourishment to the womb and fetus.

As regards intercourse, during the first trimester she may prefer to go on top to control the depth and avoid triggering heartburn or indigestion. During the second trimester, lying on her back may cease to be a good idea, so use side or seated positions. In the last weeks, when backache can be a problem, she may want to be on all fours, taken from behind or *flanquette* (*see* page 166). Sex toys are fine so long as they are clean and not used forcibly – do with them anything one would do with loving hands, tongue, or penis. Anal sex should be avoided or taken with even more care and attention than usual to avoid tearing and subsequent infection.

When it comes to the birth process, the thought of including sex may raise eyebrows, but some midwives suggest intercourse to bring on labor; once that starts, the mother-to-be can also masturbate to climax as a pain reliever. There is surely a satisfying symmetry to including the pleasure that began conception within the end result.

In the aftermath of the birth, sex may be the last thing on one's mind. Fatigue, post-labor damage, hormone imbalance – and the whole bag of responsibility for a new small person – may mean that she identifies with the new mother who, when asked by the midwife about sexual activity, exclaimed, "You don't think I'm ever going to do that again!" However, after the medical thumbs-up, there is a great deal to be said for having sex even if one doesn't feel like it. It's easy to get out of the habit and, through embarrassment, postpone the day for months or years. Consider going ahead anyway, just to know it's possible. Don't forget to check out contraception – it's a myth that breast-feeding automatically ensures protection.

Be very aware of her physical – and emotional – vulnerability. To offset, try with her on top or side by side so that she is comfortable and lubricate generously. She should tighten her buttocks to protect as he slides in – he should remain steady and let her set the pace to feel in control. If she is in pain, stop; otherwise do as much as is feasible, then celebrate. Once the habit is reestablished, trust us, it will get easier and more comfortable with time.

plateau phase

If arousal is the upwards climb from not even being aware of desire to the peak of orgasm, this is the point just short of the peak when it's good to stop, look around, and be overwhelmed by the view.

It was sexologists William Masters and Virginia Johnson who coined the term "plateau phase" for the final intense stage of arousal. Climax hasn't occurred, but it's inevitable; that knowledge in itself is part of what pushes him in particular beyond the point of no return; she, meanwhile, needs to suspend the thinking at this point in order to topple.

It is possible to prolong and deepen the moment. This is not about spinning out the intercourse part; it's way too late for that. But just at the point before inevitability kicks in, try stopping all movement, even suspending breath, concentrating on the sensations completely; this is unlikely to play the first time you try it, but with practice, perhaps even alone before together, it's entirely achievable. And once you have the experience, it's impossible to forget how completely.

The alternative is to forego your plateau in the cause of the other. Focusing all attention on your partner, assuming all responsibility, doing what works for them even if it doesn't work for you; leaving them free to climax for themselves alone. The experience of having "everything around you give you its utter attention, think only of you, care only for you" is unforgettable and transformational. For which reason every lover ought to receive it and give it at regular intervals.

his orgasm

May seem a direct and inevitable process; the reality is more complex. Like her, he needs to feel safe; unlike her, if he doesn't, he can't even make a start – for him, anorgasmia kicks in at erection stage. Once started, his needs are more specific: stimulation direct to the penis, indirect to the prostate (*see postillionage*, page 172). Some can come through scrotum or nipple stimulation alone, but his orgasmic reliability is largely dependent on target.

In terms of what is needed as opposed to where, he will already have a clear idea, honed through years of self-teaching, so can easily – given opportunity and permission – offer her lessons. The only challenge thereafter will be that if his preferred route is well trodden, the temptation for both will be never to vary from that; a truly inspired partner will occasionally override the routine and skillfully take him down a different road.

The event itself is twofold – seminal fluid gathering, then ejaculated – with the first two or three contractions stronger followed by three or four weaker ones; some men then feel an aftershock. During intercourse he may automatically shift his movements to suit each phase; working solo, she can learn to choreograph her response according to what emphasis he needs.

For a stronger, more intense climax, he can train with Kegel exercises (*see pompoir*, page 188) or experiment with approaching and then withdrawing from climax (*see* holding back, page 204) to increase blood flow into the penis. The opposite, trying to avoid ejaculation (dry orgasm), is now thought to be a bad idea and to cause medical problems.

His climax usually comes with its own evidential proof, but men have been known to fake to avoid disappointing or disrespecting a partner. Just as bad an idea – and for the same reasons – as her equivalent; it denies both the chance to find out what's actually needed. If he is doing it, he should simply stop; if she suspects he is doing it, she should gently challenge.

For over-quick orgasm, *see* hair-trigger trouble, opposite. Over-slow or not-at-all orgasm or ejaculation is rarer and usually due to disease or medication (if only recent), or emotional blocks (if long term). The answer to the first issue is a medical checkup, to the second, to take the pressure off any attempt to orgasm; much as with any orgasmic blocks she may have, he needs safety and sensuousness rather than expectation and pressure.

She can sometimes underestimate how compelling his climax is and how lost in sensation he can get – she feels sidelined. He can sometimes underestimate how withdrawn from her he can seem in the throes and hence how much she will need connection afterwards. It may help both to realize that male orgasm triggers the same brain areas as those triggered by heroin use; for him, the experience is literally an all-engrossing high.

hair-trigger trouble

Alias premature ejaculation. Forget the so-called statistics on how long an average man can keep going and how long an average woman wants him to – any ejaculation that occurs before you are both ready is premature.

At the first session with a much-desired partner, 50 percent of men either ejaculate too quickly or fail to get an erection; ensure a whole night so you can try for a comeback, but don't try too hard. If you go to sleep, he will probably wake with a huge erection. If it happens consistently with a regular partner, it may be medical; prostate infections, low serotonin levels, and certain medications have been implicated. He should see his doctor.

By far the most likely cause is what's happening mentally. While over-eagerness can be delightful on occasion, it can mean an absence of enough sex to reach optimal performance. One can ward this off solo by masturbating frequently, but in the presence of all the stimuli from a real woman – particularly a much-desired partner – this can still break down. Once anxiety kicks in, it can worsen and rule out quality sex. Time to act.

Not, however, with sex-shop creams that claim to hold you back – they are simply anesthetic and take away not only his pleasure but hers too. More appealing are active strategies. He may find it helps to relax and push out – hair-trigger trouble can be caused by anal tension – while either he or she can simply squeeze the penis, thumb and two fingers below the head, to soften the stiffest of erections. A lot can be done by using a side-by-side position so that he can't thrust much or deeply.

But these are short-term solutions. Long term, he needs to relearn his response – much premature climax is caused by his brain simply blocking awareness of the signals and so not noticing that he is at the point of no return; the answer is to be more aware rather than more controlled. He should start by masturbating alone, paying close attention to the signals and stopping as soon as he senses even the first sign of approaching orgasm, letting his erection subside, then going again. Several sessions of this should result in a good sense of what to notice and hence how – and, vitally, when – to pull back, before proceeding to more of the same but with her alongside. Repeat while embracing, then with her touching, then licking. When he can stay aware and relaxed up to that point, he can try penetration, holding still inside her for timed minute intervals. The aim always is not to hold back, but rather to build his experience and confidence.

Relationship problems may be the root cause. If he is feeling angry or hurt, the temptation may be to climax and be done without even considering her – in which case, all the training in the world won't get a result. They need to talk – and probably get professional support (*see* resources, pages 276–9).

185

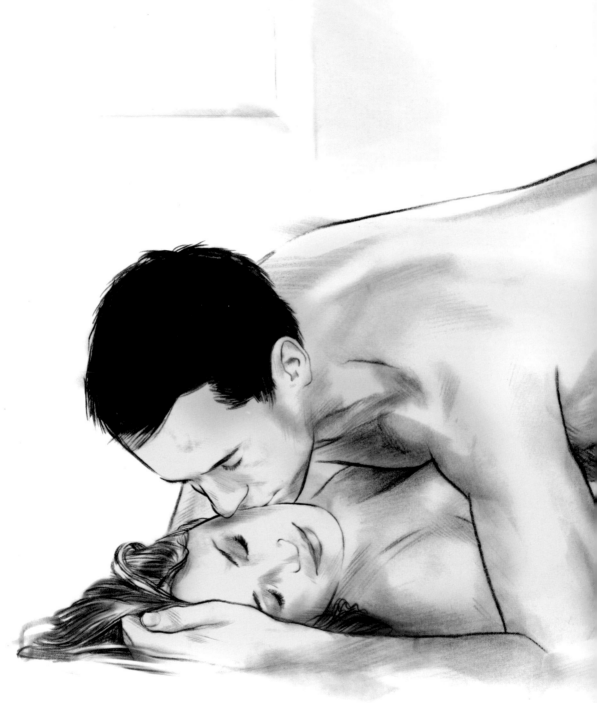

hair-trigger trouble
*either he or she can simply squeeze the
penis, two fingers below the head*

saxonus

Coitus saxonus – pressing firmly on the male urethra near the root of the penis to slow down ejaculation during orgasm. No use as a contraceptive, since sperm is around long before he ejaculates – but some women do have the knack, when giving hand work, of stopping and restarting ejaculation by urethral pressure so as to spin out the male peak.

This is best done by pressing on the shaft near the root with two or three fingers, but you need to press hard (don't bruise). The idea is to allow ejaculation to occur piecemeal. If you stop it altogether, however, he will eventually ejaculate into the bladder, which is not to be recommended. Simply slowing down ejaculation is probably harmless, but it's difficult and won't work on everyone. Women who have this technique in their repertoire say it's appreciated, but that may depend on their partner. You might as well stop just short of ejaculation, then restart the whole business a few minutes later.

pompoir

The most sought-after feminine response of all.

"She must . . . close and constrict the Yoni until it holds the Lingam as with a finger, opening and shutting at her pleasure, and finally acting as the hand of the Gopala-girl who milks the cow . . . This can be learned . . . by throwing her will into the part affected, even as men endeavor to sharpen their hearing . . . Her husband will then value her above all women, nor would he exchange her for the most beautiful queen in the Three Worlds . . . " Thus Richard Burton in his translation of the *Ananga Ranga*.

This superlative knack can be learned; traditionally, women in South India were taught it. The nearest equivalent nowadays are Kegel exercises to strengthen the pelvic floor muscles. Prescribed for urinary leaks, when done well they also develop a rippling movement in the vagina and a stronger experience of orgasm for her. She can then get to a point where she is able to draw him in and up to her G-spot (*see* trigger points, page 153), or even act as a penis ring to keep him erect after his first orgasm.

In this regard, worth perfecting. She should find the muscles that come into play when she is about to urinate, squeeze, then relax; try around two fingers to learn what it should feel like. Aim for fifty times, twice a day. Some sex-toy stores sell penis-shaped resisters to create more effective toning, though practicing with penetration by the real thing is a much better idea. He too should practice the urine-flow trick to tone and strengthen orgasm; he will feel it as a pulling up just behind his testicles. Breathe out and contract the muscle, breathe in, and release. Again, repeat multiples, twice a day.

pompoir
the most sought-after
feminine response of all

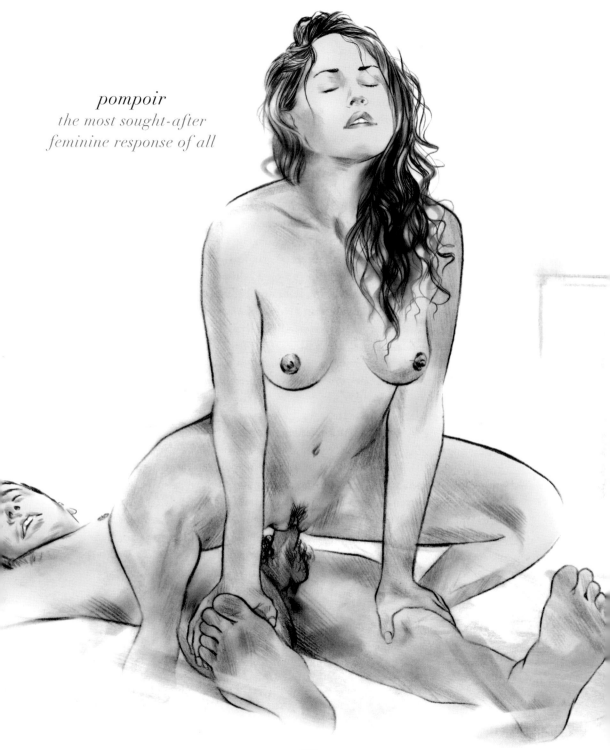

her orgasm

Unlike his, not essential for the continuation of the species. Unlike his also, often not reliable. The basic event, however, is the same: blood flowing in, a rise in tension, contractions, all with heightened breathing, heart rate, blood pressure. Given descriptions of orgasm by both men and women, expert observers couldn't identify which gender was speaking. The difference, if any, is likely to come in the symbolism. For some women the trust involved is deeply linked with relationship; not only is orgasm a sign of involvement, it creates it – hence she may be, perhaps rightly, reluctant to come with a partner she is not ready to love.

Argument rages still about the difference between the different types: "clitoral," "vaginal," "vulval," "uterine," "cervical," "blended," "G-spot." We don't think it matters where it comes from so long as it comes. We do think it matters to dispel the myth that there is one right way (*see* clitoral pleasure, page 142). To real lovers, the only question is what works for each individual her, with each individual him, in the moment.

She needs to be relaxed and unworried: neuroscientist Gert Holstege's work suggests that the fear centers of the female brain disconnect as she climaxes – and if they don't, she can't. This, as well as simple learning, is why women climax more within long-term relationships than in casual sex. New lovers may find it helps to put her in charge, dictating the moves; as trust builds, she can teach him what works and hand over control slowly.

The fact is that for most women – as for many men – hand or tongue work is the speediest route to climax. He shouldn't feel threatened by that fact – speed is much less important than quality – but take advantage of it. Watching her bring herself to her first orgasm, perhaps by vibrator, is not only arousing for him but will bring her along physically and relax her mentally. He can then follow her lead to provide her second by hand or tongue, before moving them both to intercourse (*see* bridge, opposite).

Position may be as vital to her orgasm as it is to his; experiment. Crucial will be the angle of her pelvis – some women need to arch, pushing the genitals down and away, some to tilt upwards. Given the right physiology in each partner, the CAT (*see* page 193) combines penetration and clitoral pressure; alternatively, slide a hand (or a wand vibrator) down (*see* clitoral pleasure, page 142) – easiest in rear entry or her-on-top positions.

A word about female ejaculation. If it happens spontaneously, there is no need to panic or, as one man did, sue for divorce because he thought his wife was urinating on him. If you want it to happen deliberately, the key is gentle yet persistent stimulation of the G-spot (*see* trigger points, page 153). If it doesn't happen, despite trying, her climax won't be any less pleasurable.

Two words to her about faking. Please don't. It's not only hard to do — few women can fake vaginal contractions and none can produce to order the telltale sex flush on breasts and neck — but it also sets up, in a single instant, a future of self-denial within you and deceit within your relationship. The more you fake, the harder it is to unfake — and the harder it becomes to ask for what you need in order not to have to fake in the first place. In a loving relationship, it should be possible to have an orgasm only every once in a while and still be loved.

But if once in a while is less than you want, it should also be entirely possible to remedy the situation. If she can orgasm perfectly well on her own, the clear indication is that it's about technique; this then becomes a simple matter of your both embracing the idea that what she needs in order to climax may not always be what he thinks she needs. Tell him — more important, show him.

If there is still difficulty, it's worthwhile seeing a health professional — some medical conditions and medications interfere with natural response. It may also be a good idea to consult a mental-health professional — some women's upbringing or experience of sexual trauma leave them on such full defense alert around sexual issues that climax is almost impossible (*see* resources, pages 276–9). It's always worthwhile looking at what's happening in your relationship; why should she climax with someone she dislikes, even if that dislike is trivial and temporary?

Once again, it can't be stressed enough — build a wide repertoire; the effective way may not be the same from day to day or even moment to moment. The old woman in the early Arabic sex manual *The Perfumed Garden*, whose advice to the unfulfilled couple was to try as many different methods as possible, was right five hundred years ago and is still right today.

bridge

A way to "bridge" the gap between climax without penetration and climax with it. Its origins are in sex therapy, but it has now proved adaptable for domestic use. In brief, she does whatever works for her, bringing penetration into the act more and more; over time, the two get linked and in the end the link may prove strong enough that the gap disappears.

Start face-to-face, both lying on your side or with her on top — the key is that she has room to reach down. She brings herself along by hand at her own pace, while he provides whatever additional extras she needs; his hand or her other hand keeps him erect, and at climax she switches to using his erect penis to rub her U-spot (*see* trigger points, page 153). When this is doable reliably – over a dozen sessions is remarkable progress – she starts easing down onto the penis, and climaxing with it inside, he thrusting gently if her concentration allows. The final step is for her to switch at the last moment so that his thrusts take her over the edge. Practice makes perfect and success breeds success simply through breeding confidence.

However, be warned, this technique demands expenditure on time and patience on both sides; don't get too serious about it and don't fret if it doesn't work for you. In this, perhaps as in no other game, never dance with a man you can't laugh with.

CAT
*the ultimate wish fulfillment of a
woman climaxing to order*

CAT

This has nothing to do with felines, but is an acronym for Coital Alignment Technique, one of the few ways that both partners' glans can be stimulated at the same time by penetration alone. Highly supportive to the possibility of intercourse orgasms on both sides. Probably developed by therapist Edward Eichel and team — though amusingly, when it became fashionable, a team of journalists from one of the world's foremost women's magazines allegedly claimed the credit.

He climbs on top, as in the matrimonial, but with his full weight on her; she maneuvers so that his pubic bone hits her clitoris, and as he thrusts, she tilts so that her clitoris is pulled down and then up. If that doesn't play, hand her the control. Begin with her on top (*see* upper hands, page 158), him lying still; she leans forward and experiments until she finds a position and movement that nudges her clitoris in the way she needs. Once found, he can join in by thrusting and, once perfected, they can roll over and into matrimonial; side-to-side can work too, but getting any other position to work is more or less impossible. Keep a regular yet gentle rocking rhythm.

She has to know what she wants and ask for it, even if it disrupts his pattern, so not good for men who insist there is one "right way." But if he can relax and let her take over, they may get the ultimate wish fulfillment of a woman climaxing to order.

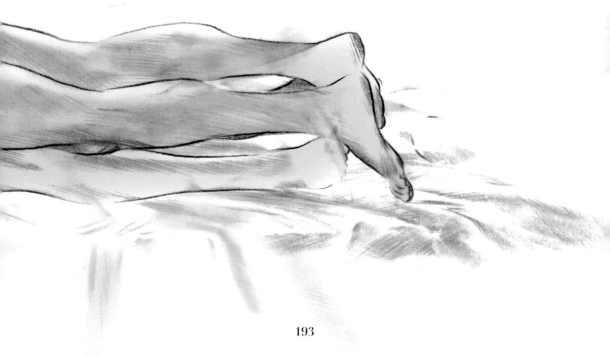

venus butterfly

Sexual pièce de résistance, originally fictional. It was invented for a plot line in a 1986 episode of *L.A. Law* as a miraculous technique to bring a woman to continuous extended orgasm, but later became an urban myth that every man wanted to know. Variously specified; the common thread is exceedingly skillful three-way stimulation of clitoris, vagina, and anus. One way might be using splayed hands with his thumb touching her clitoris, first two fingers in vagina, remaining fingers on anus; gentle opening and closing of his hands gives the "butterfly" effect. Or mouth work on her clitoris, with one or two fingers "beckoning" her G-spot (see trigger points, page 153), while the other hand probes her rectum. Some commentators — including the authors of an entire book on the subject — say it works. Others say it's physically impossible. Best to do several trial runs before a serious performance.

birdsong at morning

What your partner says in orgasm should never be quoted at them — it can be played back when you are both in a suitable mood, but only then. It's the time when people are spiritually most naked.

There is a striking consistency, over ages and continents, in what we say in orgasm. Japanese, Indian, French, and English all babble about dying ("Some of them," said sixteenth-century French historian Abbé Brantôme, "yell out 'I'm dying,' but I think they enjoy that sort of death."), about Mother (they often call for her at the crucial moment), and about religion, even if they are atheists. This is natural — orgasm is the most spiritual moment of our lives, of which all other mystical kicks are a mere translation. Men are apt to growl like bears, or utter aggressive monosyllables like "In, in, in!" The wife of the Leopard in the novel of the same name used to yell out "Gesumaria!" and there is an infinite variety of sounds short of speech.

Why these cries are so charming, it's hard to say. The Indians classified them, compared them to bird cries, and warned how easily parrots and mynahs pick them up, with bad social vibrations when they repeat the lesson — hence no parrots in the love chamber. It's important to learn to read them while enjoying the music, and particularly to know when "Stop" means stop and when it means "For God's sake, go on." This is an individual language and you need to be a sensitive field observer to learn its meaning.

Some of the "words" are common — a gasp when a touch registers right, a shuddering out-breath when you follow through. Some people talk continuously in a sort of baby whisper, or repeat four-letter words of the most unlikely kind — some you can hear several blocks away, while others still are dead silent or laugh or sob disconcertingly. Of the really noisy performers, some like to be allowed to yell, while others like to be gagged, or stuff their hair in their mouths in the style of a Japanese print (traditional Japanese houses have paper partitions). Men can be equally noisy in the run-up to orgasm, but are not usually so continuously vocal.

A naturally silent partner doesn't mean a lack of pleasure; unsurprisingly, some people still find it hard to do what – as children – they were told not to do. If you want noise, say so early on; she in particular may feel bestial when moaning or grunting, and it will help to give permission. Equally, say so if some expressions are a turnoff; there are plenty of other options (*see* words, page 99).

The important point is this: in mutual, let-go intercourse, make as much noise as you like. It's curious that we need to write this down, but house and hotel designers haven't yet realized it – they all seem to be married to noiseless, childless partners, or they would build thicker walls. Totally silent intercourse, with each partner's hand firmly over the other's mouth, can be fun if you simply can't risk being overheard.

Another variation is to have two kinds of intercourse at once – straight, gentle coitus, while each partner describes some other much wilder proceeding in fantasy, perhaps for next time. The fantasy can be as wild as you like. This is the place to experience things you can't possibly act out, and to learn your partner's fantasy needs. These fantasies can be heterosexual, homosexual, incestuous, tender, wild, or bloodthirsty – don't block, and don't be afraid of your partner's fantasy; this is a dream you are in. But be careful about recording such dreams, as they can be disturbing at the daylight level. Let them go with the release of orgasm.

Lovers who really know one another won't be frightened or take advantage. If, however, you do find this double nakedness disturbing, set rules – practicable or happy fantasies only. Never, never refer to pillow talk in anger later on ("I always knew you were a lesbian" and so on). This is contemptible. The only really disturbing manifestation of love music is when a partner laughs uncontrollably – some do. Don't be uptight about this. They aren't laughing at you.

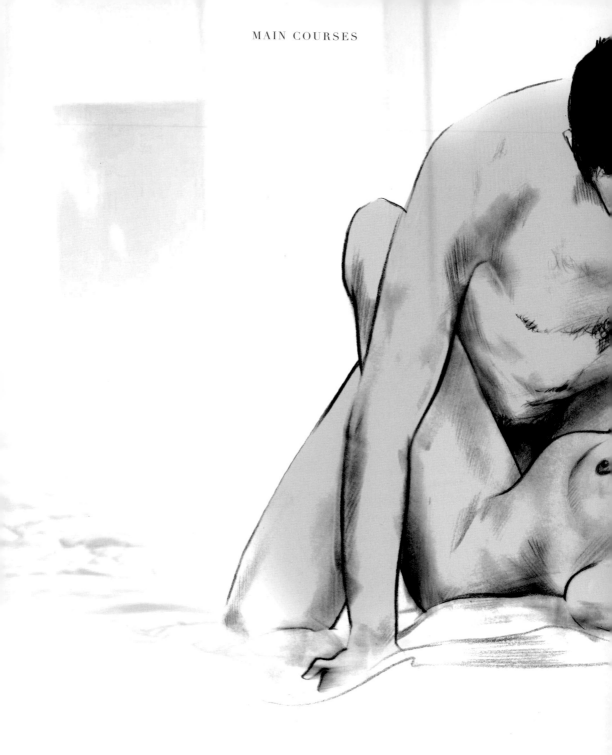

birdsong at morning
in mutual, let-go intercourse, make
as much noise as you like

little death

La petite mort: some women do indeed pass right out, the "little death" of French poetry. Men occasionally do the same. The experience is not unpleasant, but it can scare an inexperienced partner cold. One man had this happen with the first girl he ever slept with. On recovery she explained, "I'm awfully sorry, but I always do that." By then he had called the police and the ambulance.

So there is no cause for alarm, any more than over the yells, convulsions, hysterical laughter, or sobbing, or any of the other quite unexpected reactions that go with complete orgasm in some people. By contrast, others simply shut their eyes, but enjoy it no less. Sound and fury can be a flattering testimonial to a partner's skills, but a fallacious one because they don't depend on the intensity of feeling, nor it upon them.

Men can give a splendid impersonation of a fit and both sexes can also suffer instant and violent postorgasmic headaches; if symptoms occur regularly, get them checked out. In any case, you will soon get to know your partner's pattern once you are past any initial shocks. In extremis, lay them flat with legs propped up, and, if they stay unconscious for several minutes, put embarassment aside and call an ambulance.

come again
not all can, but we are sure that far more could than actually do, men especially

come again

Not all can, but we are sure that far more could than actually do, men especially. Multiple orgasm comes easily to many if not all women if they are responsive enough and care to go on, either with intercourse or hand or mouth work, after one orgasm; that is, women who definitely fall in the

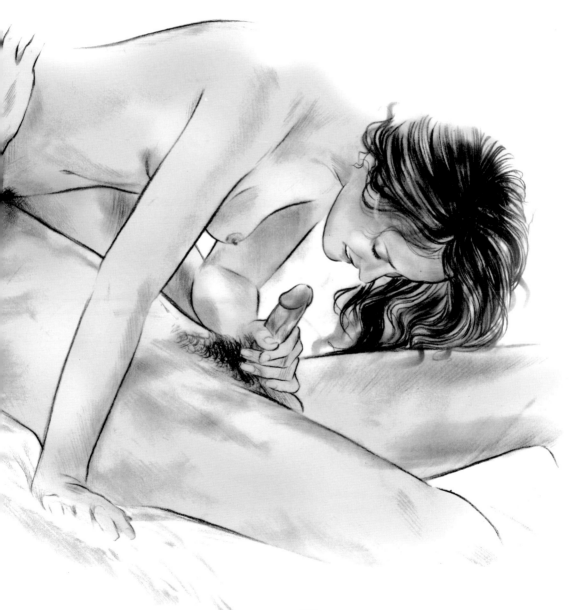

once-and-it's-over category like men do are fairly rare. Some get one continuous series of orgasms with no single, big peak. Responsiveness is beyond analysis, a subtle mixture of physiology, mood, culture, upbringing, and having the man she wants. Therefore, if she can get one really intense climax, she could probably get more if she went on. The chief exceptions are those who are fragile and tire easily, or those who want to savor the period of intense relaxation after each orgasm. If she does want to go on, the trick will be to move away from her now-too-sensitive clitoris and onto a new kind of stimulation or onto other body parts – the U-spot or urethral opening should do it (*see* trigger points, page 153).

With men it's more complicated because, like a flashbulb, the mechanics take time to come back into play again. (With a new partner it pays to establish this time early on – it may be shorter than you think; a great many men have been fooled by talk about sex being exhausting into a performance below what they could manage.) If he can't, doesn't, or is worried about it, it's no use reasoning with him. You, madam, must take over. If you look disappointed, you will have had it for the night and possibly for keeps. Suggest some diversionary entertainment, giving him half an hour, then trying to stiffen him yourself using hand and mouth work. Bring this off neatly and you will have added a new dimension to both your lives. If your ministrations really aren't working, however, pull back. Reassurance, not pressure, and a reminder that your orgasm is not necessarily dependent on his erection is what he needs here.

Two important points. One: immediately after a full orgasm some men can't stand any genital stimulation – they feel it as intense pain. If he is like this, give him a half-hour or more. Two: if he really wants penetration, quite a few women can be perfectly well penetrated with the merest half-erection if taken from behind on their side. Once started, full erection often follows.

Some men when tired get an erection that lasts indefinitely, but can't reach orgasm. This sort, who are actually slow, not fast, responders, make sexual athletes, but if their orgasm never happens, it's a medical issue and bears checking out (*see* his orgasm, page 184).

Some couples, all passion spent but still wanting one more orgasm before finishing, like to lie facing and watch one another as they bring themselves to climax. This is an added experience, not a confession of defeat, and can be immensely and unexpectedly exciting (*see l'onanisme*, pages 124–6).

excesses

Quantitatively, in sex, these don't exist – nature sees to that; the woman gets sore, the man can't go on. Medical and moral old wives have spent centuries teaching that sexual overactivity is debilitating – they were never so admonitory over excessive work or excessive exercise, and rarely over excessive eating, which is one of our most dangerous hang-ups at the moment.

Sex is, in fact, the least tiring physical recreation for the amount of energy expended. If you are flat after it, suspect either your attitude towards it, or (more commonly) secondary loss of sleep. Male lovers forget that women who work or run a home or both aren't as fresh, even though they are as willing, as the idle occupants of the old-style Ottoman seraglio. Women forget that though sex is the perfect tension relief for both sexes, preoccupation rather than physical fatigue can cause droop, especially when it goes with a wholehearted wish to perform up to and beyond Olympic standards as a matter of personal pride. Different sleep needs and sleep patterns, unrecognized and unaccommodated, can really threaten a sexual partnership. Deal with all these things by speaking out – being really in need of sleep only looks like rejection or sulking to very insecure people who can't communicate with each other.

Sex makes some languorous to the point of sedation, while others emerge boisterously productive – in the second case, get up, produce, and let your partner sleep after a suitable interval of shared quiet and love. At night there is no sleeping pill as good as violent and shared orgasm – active lovers don't need sleeping pills. If ever you do run yourself into the ground, there is no temporary exhaustion that a few hours' or days' rest won't cure.

Contrary to some belief, plenty of sex makes better and better sex – it damps down over-fast orgasm without lowering the peaks and speeds up her response: the terrific "high" after a separation doesn't depend on continence but on reunion. You can both masturbate daily while apart and still get it. Frequent sex also preserves function long into old age – not only is it a habit, but hormone levels thrive on it; so, therefore, do looks, vigor, and in particular vaginal tone. Health benefits also include reduced risk of heart disease, an immune-system boost, and a lower risk of depression. What's not to like?

One warning only: be careful if he is under the influence of the "little blue pill" – taken to serious extremes, too much activity can lead to scarring or priapism (*see* his erection, page 148). And while there is no such thing as too much sex per se, there is such a thing as too much done for too many wrong reasons, with too many wrong people – sex addiction. If sex is compulsive, driven, abusive, followed by shame and pain rather than fulfillment and joy, you need professional help (*see* resources, pages 276–9).

simultaneous orgasm

Traditional sexologists made it aspirational: Wilhelm Reich said that it made orgasm more intense; Kinsey suggested that it was the ultimate in couple intimacy; contemporary gynecologists hint that it's one way to raise the chances of pregnancy – her orgasm draws up his sperm.

In reality, simultaneity usually happens more through coincidence and luck than good management. The difficulty here is the pull between concentrating on one's own pleasure (to get you there) and concentrating on the other's pleasure (to get them there); the balancing act can push either or both of you into "spectatoring," cutting off from sensation. In sum, not an easy tightrope to walk.

Couples who know each other's movements well can try focusing on the typically "slower" partner, getting them up to speed, then leaving them simmering, so to speak, while the other catches up. Mutual hand work or *soixante-neuf* (*see* page 143) can help to get both to the edge before intercourse, and then the challenge will be to hold him back while she overcomes the classic dip at penetration and catches up with him again. The CAT (*see* page 193) may be your best option. Remember too that simultaneous doesn't necessarily mean penetrative – it's not cheating to masturbate together, nor does it preclude letting her warm up with several climaxes while he reserves his for her most reliable one.

There is an entertaining linguistic joke that the letters of "simultaneous orgasm," when suitably rearranged, read "a single amorous must." But it definitely isn't a must. Most couples never achieve it, so if you haven't, don't give yourself a hard time.

quickies

Short and sharp has a charm of its own, but it needs a rate of mutual turn-on and physical response in the woman, which is learned as a rule only in much longer sessions. A really good couple can manage either at will – short and sweet, or indefinitely prolonged and differently sweet. In other words, you can't fully appreciate the virtues of the quickie without mastering the art of prolongation.

Once you have got this, the quickie is the equivalent of inspiration, and you should let it strike lightning fashion, any time and almost anywhere, from bed in the middle of the night to halfway up a spiral stair: anywhere that you are suddenly alone and the inspiration is bilateral. Not that one or the other won't sometimes specifically ask, but the inspirational quickie is mutual; half the fun is that the preliminary communication is wordless

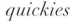

quickies
let it strike light-
ning fashion, any
time and almost
anywhere

between real lovers. The rule is never to resist this link-up if it's at all possible – and with quickness, wit, and skill, it usually is. This means proficiency in handling sitting, standing, and other postures, as well as in making love without undressing.

The ideal quickie position in terms of speedy climax, the nude matrimonial, will often be out. This may mean you have to do it on a chair, against a tree, in a washroom. If you have to wait and can go straight home, it will keep up to half an hour. Longer than that and it's a new occasion. Around the house, try not to block, even if you are busy.

holding back

Building tension to unbearable dimensions by raising, then lowering, the arousal level. Works in psychological terms by creating uncertainty and in physical terms by allowing more blood flow and so a stronger climax.

Classic arousal involves pushing ahead, keeping rhythm constant, building stimulation steadily; this is the reverse. When excitement builds, deliberately change what's happening so that progress dips temporarily in preparation for a higher peak. Most straightforward is to vary the rhythm (change stroke or keep it regular, but slow down or speed up); stopping completely is more effective, but demands more precision. Some women who like irregularity can't get there any other way.

This is a cooperative venture. Gaze into each other's eyes or listen for small shifts of breathing to gauge when to slow, when to stop, when to go on. He may break off thrusting, or she can signal him to do so, and either may halt hand or tongue. A variation is to agree that whatever happens you won't climax until permitted – or until the timer goes, or until the CD track ends. Then the tension is built from within as, together and separately, you try to surrender to the sensation without letting it overwhelm you.

Vajrayana Buddhism reputedly recommends this for both parties as a mutual path to spiritual enlightenment; it would be good to know more, but the specifics are, sadly, shrouded in secrecy. For the one-way make-'em-beg version, *see* slow masturbation, pages 269–73.

relaxation

It is probably the general experience, and we have been assuming here, that maximum feeling in orgasm goes with maximum muscular tension. A great many techniques – *ligottage* (*see* pages 252–3) and so on – are designed to boost this tension. On the other hand, it is by no means universally true. The orgasm of total relaxation is rather harder to manage, largely because it can't be boosted artificially, but is both different and, when it works, overwhelming. There are also some people, chiefly women, for whom tension seems actively to interfere with full response and too much activity seems to cause a short-circuit cut-out of arousal.

There are writings about this that suggest, for example, that tension orgasms represent fear of full release, pain, and so on. In fact, the only universal generalization about sex seems to be that no one pattern fits everyone. How far these differences between people depend on physiology is not a practically important question – some need one and some the other. Our point is that with practice most people can widen their repertoire by learning to use both tension and relaxation, and sense the needs of the moment so as to alternate them, thereby doubling their range of physical sensation and making sex still more communicative. Certainly, some tension represents fear of letting go, and some people prefer to be "forced," voluntarily, to accept orgasms – in this case, initially at least, it's probably sensible to make use of the responses you have. If you include this kind of reaction, however, don't forget to try the other mode.

The straight, sleepy, non-special intercourse, on your side or in the matrimonial position, is relaxed, but this isn't what we mean. In going for a fully relaxed orgasm, either one partner is totally passive and the other a soloist, or both achieve a state of non-effort in which wholly automatic movements - internal, for the woman – take over. Try both kinds – it's easier initially to work up both modes together.

Probably the best method at first is for the less-active partner in ordinary intercourse (this usually but not always means the one underneath) to try stopping all movement just as the orgasmic buildup begins and go completely limp (warn your partner first). Some people do this naturally: if you have had any relaxation training, starting by letting one finger get heavy and so on, use the same technique here.

You may find that on the first few occasions the fact of trying produces a different sort of tension, but after a few attempts, most easily stimulated people can learn to let their orgasm happen, and will find that this feels different from the equally pleasant orgasm one produces either by trying, or by struggling and postponing. Don't postpone – don't, in fact, be active at all. Practice the same kind of relaxation while your partner masturbates or sucks you. (For her, it may work better to try hand and mouth work first and move to intercourse only when you have mastered the relaxation approach.) The movements he or she makes will be physically the same as for "slow masturbation" (*see* pages 269–73), but the operator is looking for quite different feedback – in that "hard" version, whether the partner is tied or free, you are deliberately holding back or forcing them on, keeping just that much out of step with their reactions. In this "soft" version, you need to be a fraction ahead of those reactions so that they don't need to move, respond, or struggle. The difference can't be described, only felt. It may mean a quicker, steadier stimulation rhythm – no slow teasing and no sudden bursts – you are doing it and they are letting it happen.

Once you have got this right in intercourse and in other kinds of stimulation, including all the extras we have mentioned, you can go on to "motionless" coitus. It won't, of course, initially be entirely motionless, but see, after the first round of gentle movement, what happens if you stop thinking. Movements of a sort will continue, but in time and with practice get less and less voluntary, especially if the woman has good vaginal muscle control (*see pompoir*, page 188). Ultimately, some people learn to insert and do nothing, but still reach an orgasm in which they totally fuse, giving the sensation of being a single person – not describable, again, and probably not always realizable, but fantastic when it happens.

We should stress that this doesn't involve going slow, holding back, or any other voluntary intervention. If you find it not working, switch back to ordinary movements, but without taking too much thought – sometimes you will both sense that the moment has come to shift position and go all out for a big one; complete fusion isn't biddable, and ordinary, athletic sex is fine. If, on the other hand, it does happen, the sensation is so extraordinary you will want to repeat it.

Reliable relaxation, and the almost frightening self-loss that goes with it, are what most sexual yogis have aimed at. Some of these sexual mystics are said to recommend a special relaxed posture (man on his left side, woman on her back at right angles, knees drawn up, legs bridging his hips, feet flat on the bed). Whether this helps may well depend on your build – though it's unclear quite how to achieve penetration at this angle. What is worth suggesting, even for people who can't totally let go, is that they play through all the techniques we have described, aiming at relaxation instead of maximum tension and adjusting their feedback accordingly. Similarly, people who naturally relax in intercourse should try occasion-

206

ally to play it for full tension – just as people who like to thrash around should sometimes try being forcibly held still, and vice versa.

This sort of experimentation against one's built-in response is better value in widening one's range of lovemaking than mechanical variations of posture or trying out gadgets and stunts. It's one part of lovemaking that requires effort beyond mere curiosity, but it's essential if you hope to go as far in sexual communication as you are physically and mentally able.

afterwards

It was the philosopher Alan Watts who commented that orgasm is a delightful punctuation in the act of making love. It is not, however, a full stop, even if neither of you is able to or wants to carry on. A gentle untwining and separation, please – if penetrating, he should leave as he entered, respectfully – followed by a mutual concentration on each other to honor what has just taken place.

Physiology can both help and hinder. A cocktail of postcoital hormones can make both of you feel close and affectionate, or leave him poleaxed and her emotionally needy (*see* hormones, page 40). Tears here, the classic post-coital *tristesse*, are not usually a sign of real sadness or anxiety, but rather of vulnerability and a need to be close. The hormone prolactin can also signal to brain and body that the job is done and it's time to turn attention elsewhere; hence after intercourse in particular he may feel a strong inclination to withdraw in more than one meaning of the word. This is one time when he should override his instincts and instead give her strong, close physical contact and a few sentences of love talk. She can help by trusting that after that, silence or sleep isn't rejection.

If she hasn't climaxed, this would be the time for her to do it solo; a gentleman at this point offers either to oblige or to hold her attentively while she obliges. An arm under her head – or if she likes to be controlled, a hand pinning down her free wrist – along with undistracting touches and murmurs show that his focus is completely on her; she needs to know that her arousal is arousing him in turn. This could lead to another bout. If not, after her climax all the above notes come into play.

waking

She says: "It's the man who wakes with an erection, but women can be woken by a vaginal ache – and it's rewarding for either to be able to turn to a receptive partner. But sleep patterns matter, and while it's great to be woken in the middle of the night with intercourse, this doesn't apply when one has had a ghastly day and has an interview coming up the next morning; use some sense. It also doesn't apply in the middle of a dream one has to finish." Some people take minutes or hours to wake up, and though she can enjoy gentle intercourse waking – and it works far better than an alarm clock – don't expect athletics. The trouble is that this is the time when many males are ready for action and expect to be ridden, masturbated, sucked, and what have you. Keep these early waking workouts for Sundays and holidays, and preferably make coffee and brush teeth first,

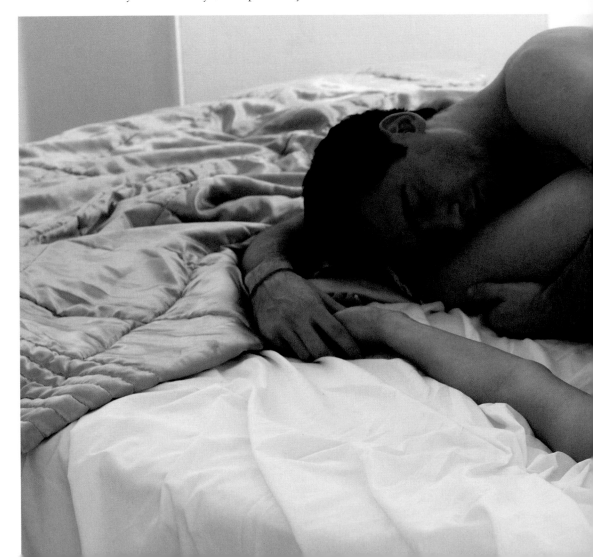

erection or no erection. Some people are lucky in having roughly the same sleeping hours, but if one were an early bird and the other a night person, that too could well give rise to real problems. If you have these, talk about them; some people do use sleep as an excuse for avoiding intercourse, but between lovers who are on different clocks it can be real and doesn't imply rejection.

If you have children, you have to be ready to be woken by them, and restrict yourselves accordingly (*see* priorities, pages 101–2).

waking
it's rewarding to be able to turn to a receptive partner

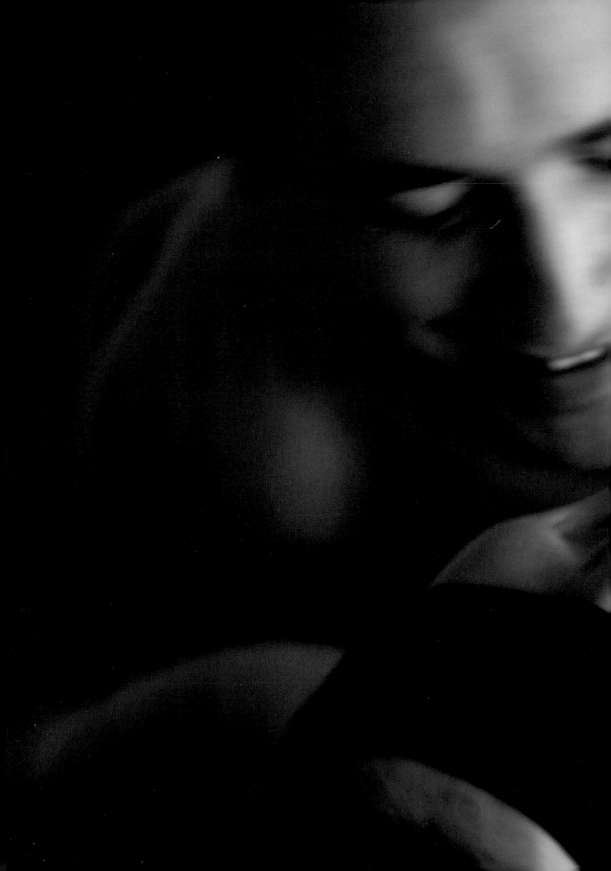

sauces and

pickles

playtime

We have said this before, but we repeat: sex is the most important form of adult play. If you can't relax here, you never will. Don't be scared of role-play. Be the Sultan and his favorite concubine, the burglar and the maiden, even a dog and a currant bun, anything you fancy for the hell of it. Take off your shell along with your clothes.

A few people are immensely excited by having sex with the assistance of the oldest human dramatic expedient – a mask – which suppresses you and makes you someone else (*see* masks, page 231). Most of us can learn to make the same change without it, and when this comes, the complete mental

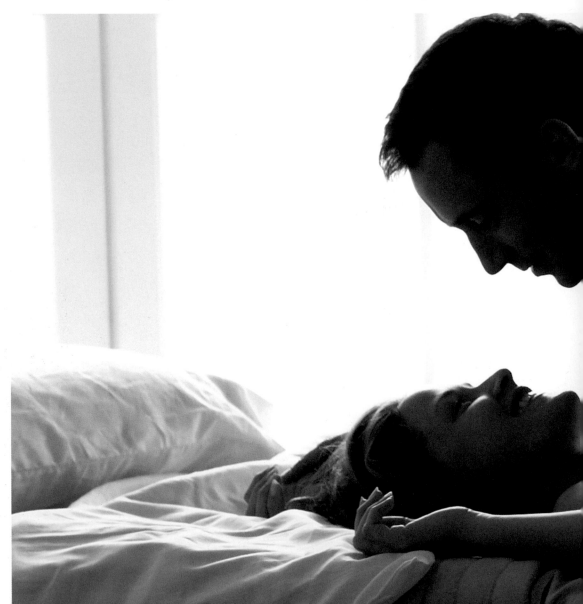

nakedness between you is the most exhilarating sort of nudism – so complete that one is healthily scared of it at first. Getting unscared is probably the most important lesson of sex. Don't use alcohol for this – it's a neutering drug. Real sex release, when one achieves it, is what drugs and alcohol are inadequate substitutes for.

playtime
take off your shell along with your clothes

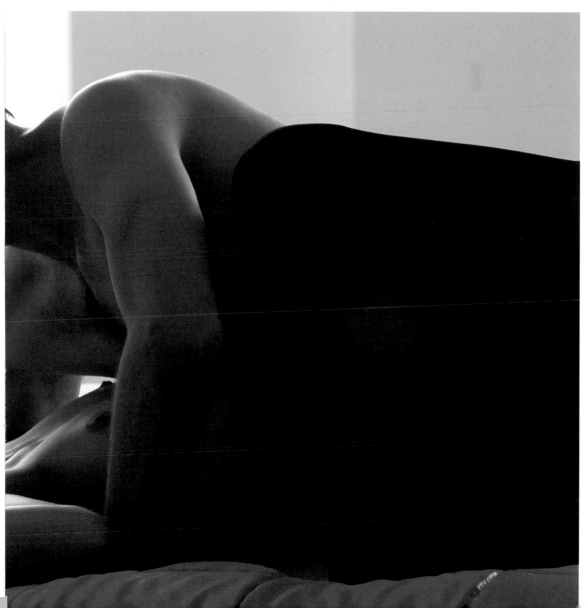

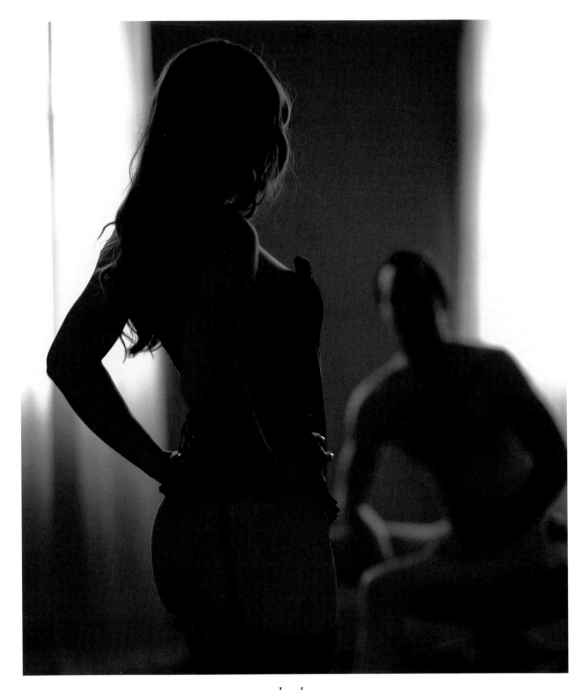

clothes
if your partner has a preference you can meet, you are unstoppable

Other turn-ons are textures — wetness, fur, rubber, plastic, leather. Many people respond slightly to all, and this is another basis of sexual fashion. Some people respond so strongly to a few that they don't hit full sexual function without them (*see* fetishes, pages 232–3). But the selection is highly individual and to tie your fly you have to know your salmon. Every such lure typically has several layers — tight, shiny, black leather is a superskin with a womany smell; it also suggests acceptance of the forcefulness of sex. Tiny, tight G-strings stress but hide her pussy, hold her perfume so she can be kissed through them, and suggest wicked, sexy girls rather than chaste sister figures. Corsets make her hourglass-shaped and suggest tightness and helplessness. And so on. A horse, seen from behind, is a "releaser" for men — it has long hair, big buttocks, and a teetering walk. A cow isn't.

Many woman have similar turn-ons themselves, but some tend to be wary of them as weird, and, in particular, to feel "he's in love with gloves or black lingerie, not with me." This is the wrong approach for either sex. If your partner has a physical turn-on, it has nothing to do with their valua tion of you, and they will love you more the more skillfully you sense and use it; hence you can catch your favorite fish at every cast. Don't try to turn yourself into something you are not — you need to feel comfortable when responding to your partner's turn-ons — but if he or she has a preference you can meet, you are unstoppable. The "you" part is in letting them see you sense it and meet it. If you too have turn-ons, say so and use them.

So, if he likes you to look like a cross between a snake and a seal, wear what he gives you, at least sometimes. If you like him a particular way, see that he knows it. Some women are bothered that a man who occasionally likes them to dress him in their clothes is unvirile (it causes less anxiety the other way round). But all of us have a person of the opposite sex inside us — Queen Omphale dressed the hero Hercules in her clothes, and he wasn't exactly unvirile. This is a common game or ceremony in other cultures. We accept sex as pleasure and are starting to accept it as play. Now we need to accept it as ceremony, plus the fact that we are all bisexual and that sex includes fantasy, self-image, role-play, and the other things that our society still finds worrying. Bed is the place to act these things out — that is one of the things human sex is for (*see* playtime, pages 212–14).

Clothing that maintains continuous sexual excitement is an old human expedient, and well worth experimenting with. Most of it is designed for women, not especially out of male chauvinism but simply because of the difference in physiology: a continuous turn-on enhances the woman's eventual response yet would tend to overload the man's and make him peak too quickly and so unable to perform long term. The traditional instances are geared to feel sexy for the wearer and look sexy to her partner. Some could be helpful in relearning the proper sexual use of our skin. They range from long, heavy earrings to tight straps, corsets, and belts, rough textures (hair- and bamboo-ring shirts), ankle chains, footwear that affects the gait and presses on the instep, and thongs that fit well into the vulva.

Most turn women on by their skin and muscle effect and men by their symbolism, but some couples get a special kick if she wears something wild under ordinary clothes on social occasions when one can't go home early. Could be worth trying for men too, if only in the interest of fair shares. Continuous sexual excitement you can't stop or do anything about would make a dull event more interesting, and guarantees good lovemaking when you do get home.

Special preferences apart, it's worth knowing as much as possible about the common turn-ons because for most couples they have stunning surprise value as unscheduled extras on special occasions. If a particular one doesn't work, you needn't repeat it.

corset

An obligatory article of fashion in the past, now back as an everyday evening style that's also useful for sex games. Makes a woman still more woman-shaped. Firm pressure on the waist and abdomen excites many women. Probably works through tightness and skin pressure, but a lot of symbolisms are also involved.

G-string

No longer confined to sex shops, now widely available. It should tightly cover the whole pussy and pubic hair, nothing else. It should undo from the sides with hooks, or better still with ribbons, so that it can be taken off when astride without kicking the man. It is best made of silk, not nylon, because it holds her perfume better. Other materials can be used as turn-ons, for looks, but can't really be kissed through – if she wants to use these, she should wear them over the silk "leaf."

The sexiest G-string is one that isn't used for street wear, but reserved only for sex: the first direct genital kiss is given, or taken, through it. Later, she can surprise him by suddenly taking the two ends and putting it hard over his nose and mouth.

A variation on the G-string is the thong, which presses on the perineum; correctly worn, by him as well as her, it can leave one gasping. Open-fronted panties aren't the same thing. Edible panties are a joke, but if you must, don't simply chew them off; nibble and lick piecemeal.

shoes

High heels attract some males, maybe for their effect in increasing the wobble in the female gait, another instance of making the woman appear more woman-shaped.

That said, for most lovemaking you really need bare feet. For which purpose, to take shoes off elegantly, she shouldn't bend, but stay standing, lift up the leg behind, and remove one-handed.

boots

Notorious sex turn-on for many people – the longer the better. Complicated symbolism here involving aggression (jackboots and so on). Used to be the badge of the prostitute – now general wear for everyone: odd how the market in the respectability of sexually symbolic clothing swings over the years. One could learn a lot about human imprinting by plotting the prevalence of such preferences.

Good for dressing-up games if you like them. But a spiked heel is a dangerous weapon, so take care; hence not very practical for serious sex unless you keep them for non-horizontal, non-bed activities. If her man likes them, she should try appearing suddenly in long, tight, black shiny ones.

stockings

Can be a sex turn-on – often the preferred ones are old-style black stockings, which look extra naughty when paired with suspender belts that draw attention to the essential zone. Tights are an obstacle unless crotchless, and non-erotic in any form. It's said that if he can get one stocking off her, he is home. Actually, in quick undressing or actual lovemaking, both tights and stockings get ruined, but if you keep your nails and fingers smooth, taking them off gently makes good foreplay, along with mutual undressing generally. Long gloves turn some people on; they suggest the old-style great lady.

clothes
there to be taken off

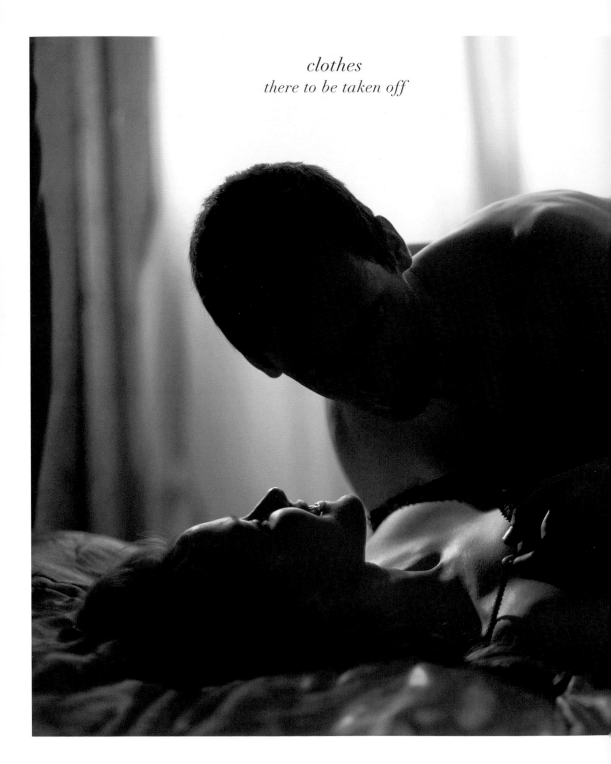

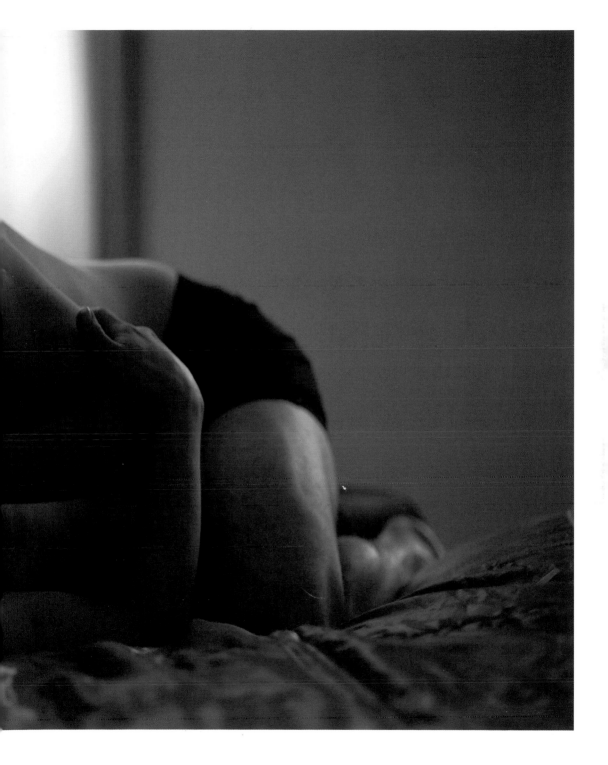

ben-wa balls

When Japanese, called *rin-no-tama*; come in various configurations designed to massage vaginal spots (*see* trigger points, page 153), from simple pairs of plastic spheres to metal balls one inside the other or those with a built-in vibrator. They can either be inserted into the vagina or put between the labia (don't insert in the anus, as they can get lost). Movement, including walking, then produces a quite unique pelvic sensation more intermittent and intimate than a vibrator. Some can be used in intercourse, others to maintain a steady stimulation — all day, if she can take it. If she can't keep them in, she should try plastic ones, which are less likely to drop. If she can't get them out, she should take a deep breath and bear down. Useful for strengthening pelvic floor muscles (*see pompoir*, page 188).

boutons

Any device — often a penis ring — worn over his pubis and providing an additional pressure point for the clitoris. One particularly fine specimen was described in the first edition of this book as "Chinese and made of ivory (with) two sky-dragons . . . sporting with a pearl (the semen) — in use, the pearl is a small knob to fit the clitoris, the scales of the dragons open and tickle the labia, and the whole thing is held in place by a long tape passed through a hole, back between the legs, crossing behind the scrotum, up between the buttocks and then round the waist."

Jelly plastic has now solved the problems of clitoral knobs being too hard to be comfortable, and some come with vibrators. Begin with classic him-on-top positions where he rides high and can keep the vibrating part in constant contact. Then experiment; he may need to grind with a circular movement rather than thrusting.

rubber

This turns some people on, and is a whole-time fetish with others. Its effect seems to depend on its status as superskin combined with tightness and odor. The odor of latex rubber excites some people if they have come to associate it with using condoms. Rubber is difficult to clean — try washing in soapy water. Black seems to be the preferred sexual color.

leather
a turn-on that women respond to as much as men

leather

Probably the most popular superskin turn-on. Black hide also looks aggressive or scary and is the S&M textile of choice, for dominators and dominated alike; others, even if they are not into bondage, like to be encased in it or to see a partner encased. Unlike rubber, you can wear it without being thought weird, which is yet another example of the arbitrary social choice of sex turn-ons in clothing. If your partner likes it on you, let them do the buying. This is one object turn-on that women respond to as much as men, especially if it feels and smells right (*see* boots, page 221).

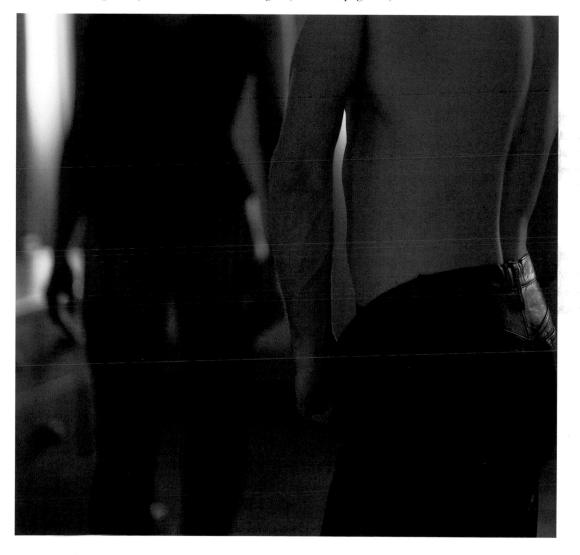

striptease

The modern version probably began in the 1890s at the Moulin Rouge in Montmartre, Paris. In one variation, a woman removed her clothes in a vain "search" for a flea. Once seen as immoral and illegal but now par for the course, strip shows, and their more hands-on sister lap-dancing clubs, may still leave a bad taste because of the possibility of performer exploitation.

It could now be her in the audience almost as easily as him; the Chippendales dancers began that shift in the early 1980s and the film *The Full Monty* completed it in 1997. For partner purposes, the important thing is to agree on boundaries before either of you proceeds. One way could be to attend a show together – with a non-breakable "we leave now" signal – and then discuss afterwards whether it's OK to go again, and whether separately or together. Variations include floor shows, pole dancing, peep shows, and private dancing monitored by ceiling camera; if you want actually to touch,

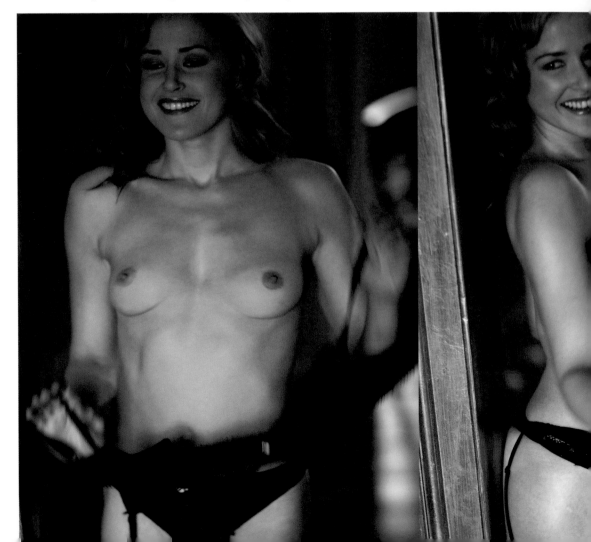

choose the more rowdy audience-participation events aimed at girls' or stag nights, or go to a lap-dancing club where, for the length of one song, she will rub up against you. New Burlesque is the up-market, cabaret version with expensive fin-de-siècle, choreographed poses and a strictly hands-off policy.

When stripping for each other, it's the performance of Burlesque that's most easily copied and most elegant. A magnificent prelude to lovemaking, particularly when she offers it as a gift to him – "tease" here is the operative word. She needs attitude for this, head high, breasts out, hands running along body contours to direct "audience" attention. Keep eye contact.

striptease
a magnificent prelude to lovemaking

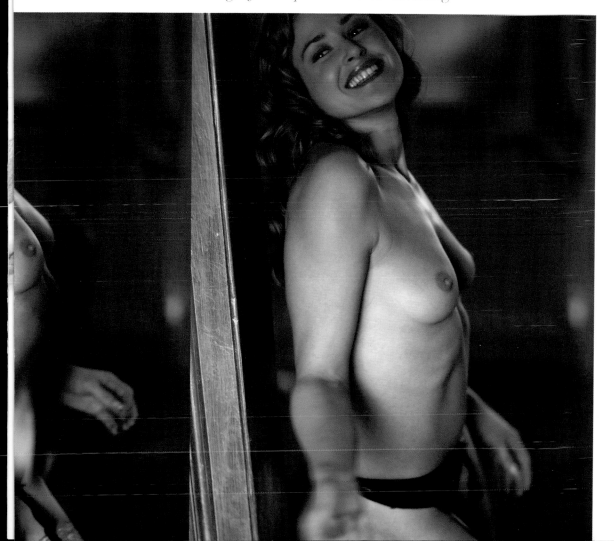

jokes and follies

Sex, contrary to cultural traditions among prudes, is preeminently the right place for these. The best jokes too tend for this reason to be at the prudes' expense. The finger-raising quality of lovers vis-à-vis society is as necessary psychologically as their tenderness to each other. That, and not just the spice of danger, is what makes love in odd places and under other people's unperceptive noses so attractive. This is childish, but if you haven't yet learned to be childish in your lovemaking, you should go home and learn, because it's important.

One mustn't let the joke go wrong and sour things: if you can have inter-course in a public restaurant or on Auntie's dining table and bring it off, you can laugh about it after (but if you don't bring it off, you will be lucky if you speak to each other again). Most couples contain, for any given occasion, one danger lover and one restraining influence, and achieve accordingly a common-sense balance, helped by the angel who watches over such lunatic antics and protects lovers from the consequences. All in all, it would be stupid to recommend them, but a pity to have missed them.

The amount of laughter you have in intercourse, pranks apart, is a measure, we think, of how well you are managing to love. It's evidence for, not against, the seriousness of your communication. If you have this, the laughs never fail, because sex is funny. If you haven't, you end with boxed ears or tears or no orgasm all around, through some remark "destroying the atmosphere." When it's really going, laughter is part of the atmosphere – even mockery isn't unaffectionate, though you should never laugh at, only with, and there is no joke like love well and mutually completed under unlikely circumstances. It's one of the few contemporary occasions that gets a laugh out of pure joy.

Taking a partner (usually female) round to social occasions nude, or in some sexy gear, under a long coat is a game that some couples relish. It can be dangerous – if you must do it, make sure she really enjoys it. The no-panties bit is on the whole dangerous enough for most women unless it's very much their thing.

jokes and follies
laughter is a measure of how
well you love

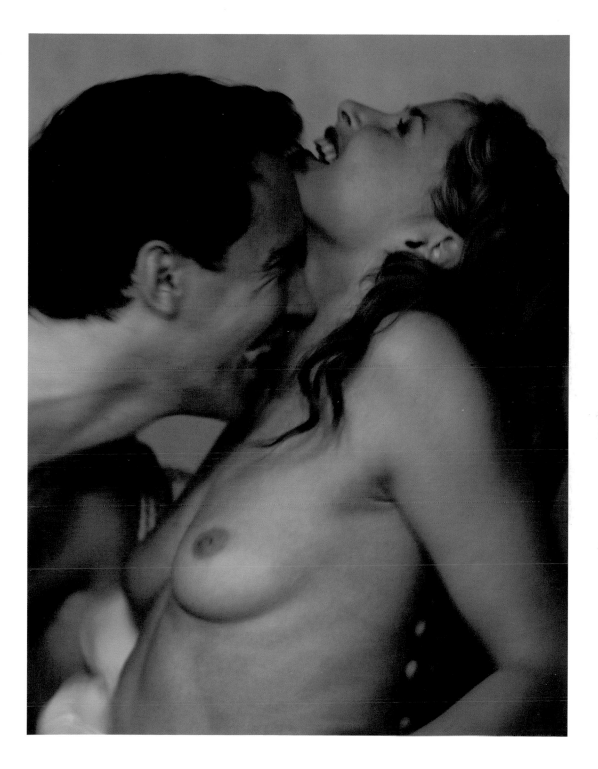

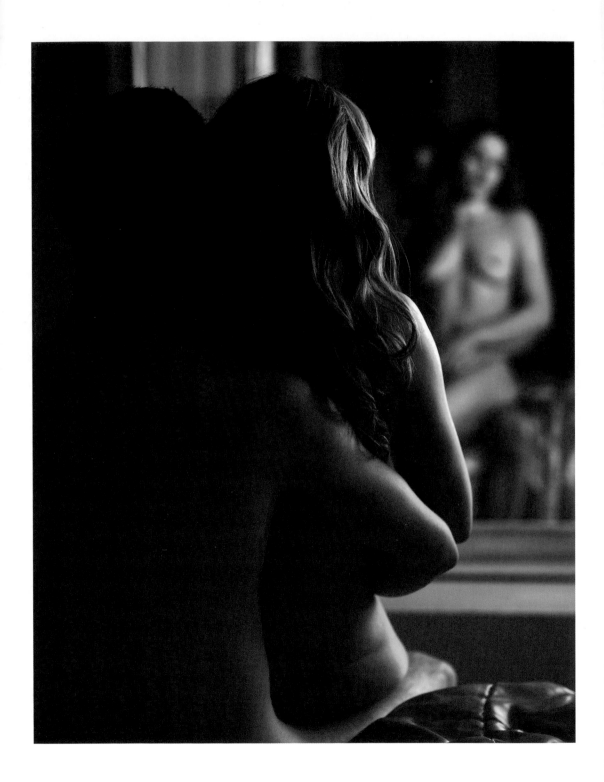

mirrors

These have always been an important part of sexual furniture in any bedroom not wholly devoted to sleeping. They turn lovemaking into a viewing occasion without loss of privacy and help it progress at a practical level. They also provide a turn-on by letting you see yourselves – he can see his own erection and movements without stopping. She may be turned on by seeing her own body, watching herself masturbate, seeing herself bound, or any of the other fantasies one can enact, so that both experience viewer as well as participant pleasure.

Those who don't like them, by contrast, say they spoil the shut-in, non-spectator feeling they need to appreciate sensation to the full, and make the bedroom less like a womb with twins in it and more like Tiffany's. Plus it must be said that the feelings of exposure mirrors bring may make her in particular struggle with internal insecurities that she is not as magnificent as the current media icons, who – we too often forget – have been enhanced by specialist lighting and computer magic. Loving and genuine fascination with her body is the best way to silence her self-doubt.

If you have never made love in front of a big mirror, try it. You really need more than one to enable both of you to see clearly without having to shift around. The exercise is worth it, not only for voyeur effect but to show you how unridiculous you look making love. Sex described in cold blood, like instructions on how to put up a deck chair, sounds undignified, but seen as one participates, it is natural, attractive, and formally beautiful to a morale-boosting extent. If there does come a time when it's better to feel only, and never look, we haven't reached it yet.

Old-style brothels went in for rooms of a hundred mirrors. Expense apart, these may or may not work for you; a hundred couples acting in unison may be your turn-on, or they may remind you of Red Square on May Day or a Roman orgy rather than lovemaking.

mirrors
turn lovemaking into
a viewing occasion

trains, boats, planes

Railways were an old and favored site for "different" sex — now hardly possible given new-style open compartments, except possibly in sleeper cars when there are only two of you. Whether it's the motion and acceleration or the association with love on the run that provides the turn-on isn't clear: it's said that the classier Parisian and Viennese bordels used to have a compartment fitted up, complete with train effects and noises, and vibrated by a motor and cams. Since it's probably the motion that scores, choose a hard couch, and a winding track with numerous intersections and switches. In emergency, there is just enough room for an upright in the washroom.

More usual nowadays — and also dependent on washroom use — is sex on planes. Otherwise known as the Mile High Club — whose founder, Laurence Sperry, inventor of the autopilot, once emerged naked from a crash landing in water along with his female passenger; the ensuing headline read: "Aerial Petting Ends in Wetting." The rush with air travel may be due to the vibration, the lower atmospheric pressure increasing orgasmic intensity, or simply the illicit nature of it all. If desperate and unwilling to go the washroom route, one can work wonders with wandering hands under strategically placed airplane blankets and a tolerant cabin crew.

Boats, despite the challenges of instability, offer huge possibilities; big ships have private cabins; small ones can be sailed away to remote locations.

cars

These approach the ideal form of locomotion, the "double bed with an outboard motor." Big old cars come very close to it (there is room to lie flat, even on the rear seat). Current smaller machines call for neat handling of anything more than breast-and-petting work. The classical postures (she on the backseat, he kneeling between her legs, or both sitting, her legs around his waist) were developed for use by Madame Bovary in hansom cabs. All cars, whether adapted to petting or coition, can be goldfish bowls unless you live in a climate where the windows quickly mist over. If you rely on condensation, it's nevertheless a good idea to have a powerful light ready to dazzle potential prowlers.

For alfresco love, the least-screened parking site is the safest, like a French eighteenth-century bower, because you can't be crept up on. Remember, however, that in most countries motorvehicle action visible from outside can earn perpetrators a stern police warning, or worse (*see* voyeurs, page 246). If you want to do much of this, buy a small van, or one of those mini-campers known as adultery wagons, which are in effect

242

mobile houses. It takes confidence to strip naked in any of these. Mutual masturbation while on the move, and trying to score the number of orgasms per gallon, are popular fantasies, but against both the law and the interests of safe driving. For those who like restraint, seat belts can be worn or you can tie one party to his or her seat and approach your work slowly.

open air

Countries with a warm summer have advantages that can't be overstated. In England, to have regular and full love outdoors, you need to be frost-proof and own a park. In Ireland or Spain, even though it's warm in Spain, you need to be priest-proof as well. Most parts of the USA should count their blessings in this regard. What is odd is that they don't do more about garden design. The walled or hedged gardens of Europe are nearly all practicable, at least by night.

Outdoor locations in wild areas are often flawed by vermin, ranging from ants and mosquitoes to snakes and officious cops. Nevertheless, respect flora and fauna. Don't ejaculate – or anything else – without clearing up after yourself, and never in natural water sources. Also remember that discarded condoms can kill the wildlife.

Surface-wise, the best venue is often sand dunes, which give shelter and keep the heat, besides not harboring stinging insects. Lawn grass is fine if well screened. The safest cover, if you intend to strip right off, is the thicket standing on its own, where you can see out, but they can't see in; the "bower" of Fontainebleau painters. Europeans, who live in crowded landscapes, are adept at quick dressing and using places such as Hampstead Heath and the Prater.

With so many landscape opportunities to choose from, there should be no problem finding somewhere appropriate – if you do take risks, however, cultivate the quick getaway; danger turns some people on, and others, of both sexes, right off. Enthusiastic larks one gets lost in, like stripping right off or tying each other to trees, call for very remote areas or a walled garden.

Even more crucially, check out local customs and laws, particularly religious mores, and be respectful of them – otherwise you risk both offending local feeling and incurring serious penalties. The many ethical systems in the world view sexual display in different ways, and an affectionate kiss, in some countries, is a deadly insult to deeply held beliefs. A flat roof at night is a standard Eastern venue – you can make love and see the whole city.

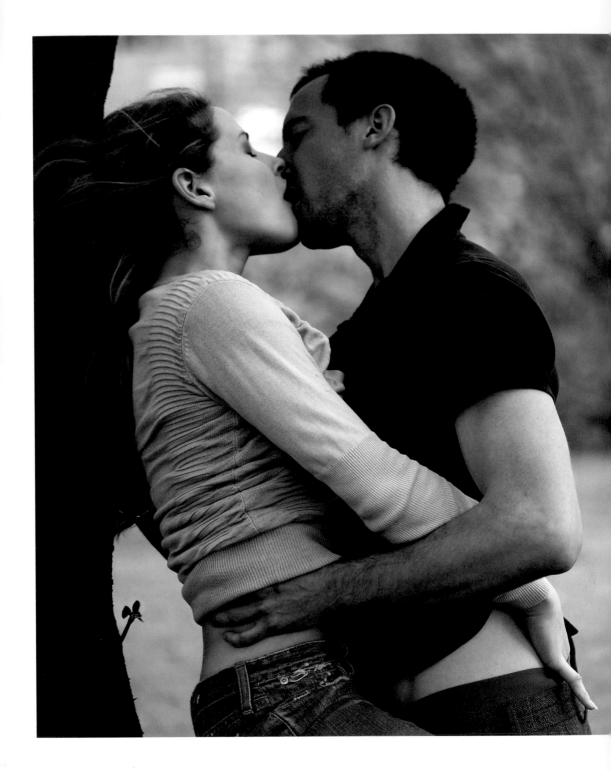

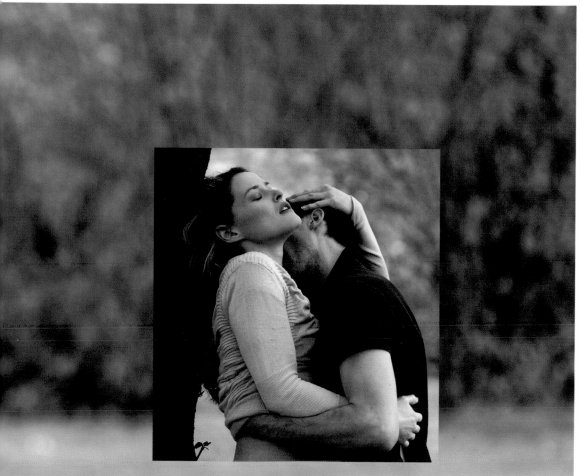

open air
enthusiastic larks call for
very remote areas

remote control

It's an old story that you can seduce a complete novice, who has no idea what you mean, by slipping a thumb into a closed fist, or between your lips, and absent-mindedly moving it in and out, in and out. Frankly, however, most people this works on know very well what it's all about.

The lip one works better, nail downwards in the appropriate rhythm — she will feel it where she should. She can do the same "at" him, for example in eating. Once habituated to either of these signals, most women and some men can be radio-controlled as to excitement, erection, and even orgasm — even by rubbing the lobe of one's ear — from several places down a table, the opposite side of a room, or the opposite box at a theater. One very humorous use of this was when the lady was dancing with someone else, who spotted what was going on in his arms and thought he was the source of the signals — which actually came from her lover, who was sitting out.

Nowadays, more literal and technological remote control, prefigured by the Pleasure Machine in *Barbarella* and the Orgasmatron in *Sleeper*, is an everyday reality: vibrators triggered by mobile phone, teledildonics for Internet pleasuring, and so on. Given the distance at which some people now have to conduct relationships, it's more than likely just the beginning.

voyeurs

Title to be kept for those who treat sex as a non-playing spectator sport. Any active player is likely to be fascinated to watch their game being played, provided the players themselves are worth watching. Real couples are doubtless worth watching — the bored, semi-erect participants in blue movies, on the other hand, seldom merit the trouble. Real human mating behavior is as interesting as that of the birds of the air and the beasts of the field, and far more instructive.

Nowadays, however, the opportunity to watch real couples in the flesh is unusual — we keep our sex behind closed shutters. Those shutters are opened now and again via webcam coverage on "real sex" websites, as well as sexual acts in semi-public places performed for the delectation of passers-by (termed "dogging," derived from the euphemism, "Just going out to walk the dog, dear"). These, though often illegal, at least contain some degree of genuine passion.

Shutters may be necessary, for the protection of individuals as well as in the interests of social comfort. But we lose a lot in this society by not being in the habit of making love in company. If we did, fewer books such as this one would need to be written.

erotica

In the first edition of this book, the equivalent section was entitled "pornography," and the opening sentence was "Name given to any sexual literature someone is trying to suppress." Times have changed: what was suppressed in 1972 has now been renamed erotica and is available on the middle rather than the top shelf. The worldwide sex industry sales for 2006 were reported to be $97 billion, twice the sales of Microsoft, and targeted at both sexes.

There are still, however, some things that are unacceptable and rightly so: violent, degrading, or exploitative materials should form no part of one's repertoire and real lovers will surely join us in condemning them. Equally objectionable is when sexual material means that one partner loses confidence, or loses attention for the other, though recent research suggests that erotica use is often a symptom of depression, and thus may need treatment rather than divorce. When a spouse has no energy for post-work conversation then disappears and spends six hours surfing the net, what may need to be put on the table is what underlying mental problems have meant that for him (or her) surfing has become more attractive than love or life.

More positively, if used in context and with consensus, erotica strengthens the love bond. Depiction of any of the range of sex behaviors we describe helps people to visualize them, which is why this book is illustrated. Straight couples can use erotica constructively in the exact proportion that it's well done; that is, it describes feasible, acceptable, and pleasurable activities they would enjoy, or fantasies that, though not feasible, turn them on. Many people find sex books a real help in raising the level of feeling to bed point. She says: "Don't see erotica as a rival but as an ally; making it part of what you do will be much more likely to proof your relationship against the danger of its taking over."

First, however, choose your erotica. It isn't true that only men are turned on by sexual material; it is true that women are most turned on by it if it's written with sensitivity and an awareness of other than male feelings. Plus remember that much erotica is so idealized that it can provoke inferiority complexes on both sides; choose with an eye to self-esteem as well as arousal, or the arousal may be non-existent.

Here are some classics: the *Kama Sutra* and *The Perfumed Garden* for traditional ideas; Nancy Friday's *My Secret Garden* for a modern view; Anaïs Nin's *Delta of Venus* and Pauline Réage's *Story of O* for something more edgy. As for films, mainstream sensuality may actually be more effective than videoshop raunch, at least for her: Sharon Stone riding Michael Douglas in *Basic Instinct*; Julie Christie and Donald Sutherland making married love in *Don't Look Now*. You will have your own favorites.

blindfold

A deprivation tool, focusing attention on four senses because one is blocked; if you are tempted to think too much, this will neatly short-circuit the temptation. Traditionally, central to power exchange sex (*see ligottage*, pages 252–3); blindfolded, you don't know what's about to happen and this alone can tip some women into an orgasm. Essential is trust; never blindfold without warning or negotiation, and once blindfolded never inflict an unpleasant surprise or you will ruin more than just the moment.

A light scarf or a long-haul-flight sleep mask will act as a symbolic blindfold, but for true darkness, source a thicker one from a sex shop. With a novice, keep reassuring hands-on touch and tell them what you are doing; with a non-novice, you can raise the anxiety level with extended silences and temporary withdrawal of contact. Waft scents, offer tastes, whisper fantasies. The master sensory channel, however, is touch, administered unpredictably: move silently and slowly so there are no betraying cues. Use mouth and genitals, but also feathers, sex toys, ice, tingle creams. When the blindfold comes off, expect disorientation – time for close, safe embrace.

At the other extreme is deep eye contact; in one academic experiment a randomly allocated pair of strangers who held just four minutes' eye contact fell in love. Use your eyes not only to create a bond pre-sex, but also to hammer home the intensity during lovemaking. Keeping your eyes open during orgasm can feel almost overwhelmingly intimate.

chains

The tied-up, tinkling look – they show well on naked skin. Some women like both the coldness and the symbolism, and some men spend hours locking and unlocking them – both should try them on each other for size. Uncomfortable and only symbolically effective if you want actually to hold a partner still, but they look fierce, and some find them exciting. Bright tinkling objects turn on people as well as magpies (*see* earlobes, page 65).

harness

Quick "restraint" system for people who can't tie knots, who bruise with rope, or who like the look of "apparatus." Comes in all degrees of complication and for all postures – watch out for expensive confections that are really props for soft-core porn photos. Mainstay of fetish boutiques. Gives very tight restraint and a lot of skin pressure. Some play up the horse symbolism.

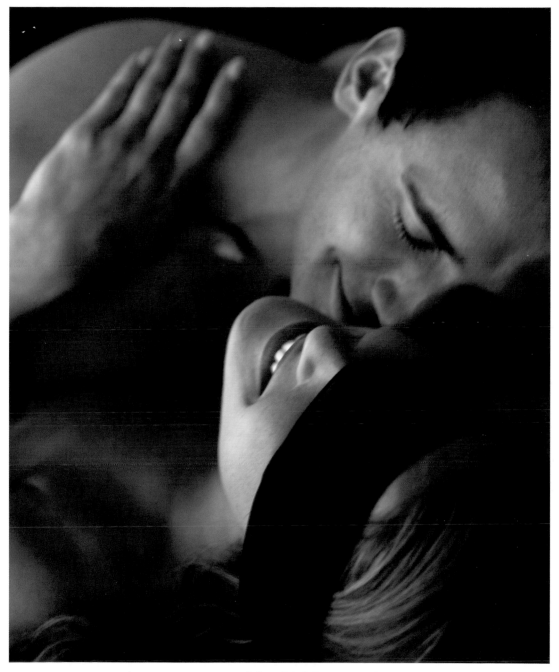

blindfold
waft scents, offer tastes, whisper fantasies

gags

Some energetic people like to be gagged. As one lady put it, "it keeps the bubbles in the champagne." Gagging and being gagged turns many on and the expression of erotic astonishment on the face of a well-gagged partner when they find they can only mew is irresistible to most. Apart from the symbolism and the "feeling of helplessness," it enables the subject to yell and bite during orgasm, which helps a total cut-loose, unless you have a rhinoceros hide and live in a soundproof room. It makes prompting impossible, so that your partner's initiatives are outside your control. Most men who are excited by this sort of game like to be silenced thoroughly. Untimid women often come to like it after a few tries if they are the biting kind or like the feeling of helplessness – others hate it and lose their orgasm; if so, don't even try. A few like to be blindfolded as well, or instead.

It's hard to gag anyone so they are 100 percent quiet except in movies, where a wisp of silk over the heroine's face enables the hero to walk past without hearing her. A long piece of cloth, with several turns well between the teeth, or the sex shop rubber ball centrally fixed in a narrow strap, is quite fierce enough. Adhesive tape will work, but is torture to take off.

The prisoner must never be made incapable of signaling if anything is wrong. Anything in the mouth must be firm, mustn't block breathing, and must be quick-release in case the subject signals danger – from choking, feeling sick, or any other source of discomfort; best not to use at all if the subject has any condition that affects breathing. The "stop signal" must be agreed beforehand and never abused or ignored (*see* hazards, pages 260–1). Penalty for illicit use, two further orgasms.

rope work

To make *ligottage* (*see* pages 252–3) work as a game, it obviously needs to be effective but not painful or dangerous. So technique is worth a few words, because some skill and care are called for.

On any bed with four posts you can stake a partner out, supported by one or more pillows. Extension like this inhibits orgasm in some people – many feel more with the legs open, but the wrists and elbows firmly behind the back, or by being tied to a chair, or upright to a post. The critical areas where compression boosts sex feeling are the wrists, ankles, elbows (don't try to make them meet behind by brute force), soles of the feet, thumbs, and big toes (artful partners break off halfway to tie these last two with a leather bootlace – if you doubt this, try it). The Japanese take this further, making rope work an art form; if it appeals, surf the Internet for full instructions.

There are divergences of taste over what to use for tying. Leaving aside extremes like straitjackets, different couples use leather or rubber straps, ribbons, cloth strips, pajama cords, bondage tape, Velcro fastenings, or thick, soft rope. Straps are easiest for those who aren't very strong, or can't tie reef knots; they need holes at intervals. Handcuffs may hurt to lie on, but can be removed fastest; for safety's sake carry them closed, and for heaven's sake keep the keys within reach. For most couples a hank of cotton clothesline is fine. Cut it into five or six lengths of about 4 feet and a couple of about 6 feet, and use a lot of hand-tight turns. Put rope through the washing machine with softener before use.

Bondage can be played without any of the props and simply for the symbolism: instructing the unbound other to lie still and "bear" whatever you are doing can have spectacular results as they struggle to reconcile the desire to respond and the contradictory injunction. On the other hand, usually at least half the payoff in people who enjoy it (and there are many) is, for the person tied, directly physical – in struggling against restraint and in skin and muscle feeling. It also helps get over our cultural taboo on intense extragenital sensations, which belongs in the same package.

Rope marks usually go in a few hours if you have been gentle. Rope burns and bruises come from clumsy untying – don't saw through the skin, but be quick so that the man doesn't get stiff through being left tied after orgasm, and the woman comes down to earth lying comfortably in your arms. You can be agreeably, adequately, and symbolically fierce, whichever your sex, without being spiteful or clumsy and wrecking things (*see* hazards, pages 260–1).

The right mix here, as in all sex games, is tough plus tender. If you can't sense how tough your partner likes it, ask, then subtract at least 20 percent to allow for the difference between fact and fantasy. Given these rules, any couple who enjoys forceful lovemaking and likes the idea could do worse than learn to make each other helpless occasionally, gently, quickly, and efficiently. This is neither weird nor frightening – just human. For the pièce de résistance that goes with bondage, namely slow masturbation, go to that section (*see* pages 269–73).

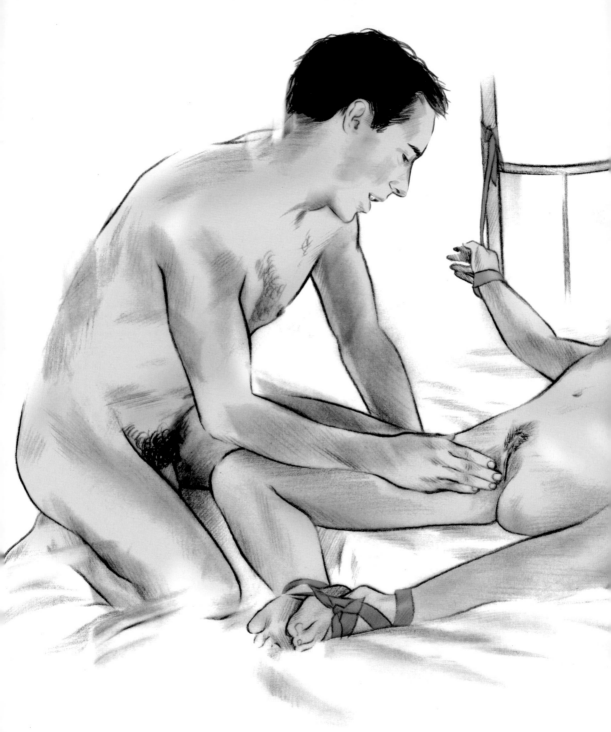

rope work
the right mix here is tough plus tender

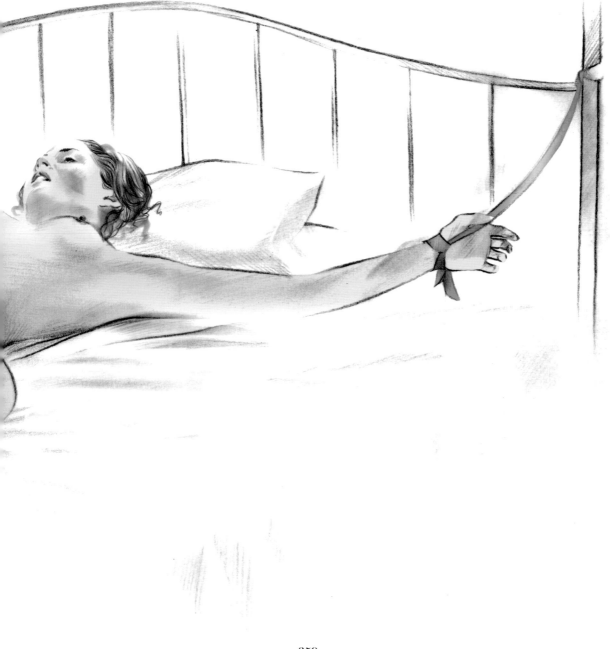

vibrators

Contrary to myth, not an embarrassing aid for the lonely or inexperienced, but vital for both solo and couple sex. They come in several varieties – penile, clitoral, G-spot, anal, egg-shaped, double, handbag-sized, fingertip, cock ring, strap-on, slip-down-your-knickers, and so on – not counting the kits that transform your cell phone or music system. Some people simply don't respond, others think vibrators desensitize or make the user dependent – but if wanted or liked, a solid relationship can surely incorporate, rather than feel threatened by, sex toys, vibrators included.

To see if they work for you, an electric toothbrush (with unused head) can act as a nursery-slope run; useful too if one forgets to pack the vibrator. Once you know what you want, visit a sex shop; the protocol for testing intensity and speed is against your nose or palm (*see* sex shops, page 249). Think about what you will be using it for and choose accordingly: G-spot vibes are curved, anal are flared so they don't disappear inside. Shape is mostly a red herring – it's the vibration not the structure that has the effect – and while he may automatically choose penis-shaped, she usually gets more benefit from a form she can easily hold and apply. If she wants to insert the device, she should check the manufacturer's instructions, since some aren't suitable. Low-speed silicone is quieter, but any can be muffled by a pillow held at groin level. Some materials can cause allergies and hormone disruption; a good sex shop can advise on current developments.

Care and maintenance: the same as for any sex toy – clean before and after, add lubrication for ease (*see* lubrication, page 65), use a condom if sharing with an untested friend (*see* safe sex, pages 96–8). Rules for use: really none – if it feels good and isn't painful, continue to do it. Incorporate into the ritual of skin stimulation, then home in on lips, nipples, bottom cheeks, and the small of the back on either side of the spine before moving on to genitals proper.

Traditionally, the vibrator is her instrument – she can use it to show him what she needs, or to take her first orgasm solo as a warm-up. Holding the vibrator firmly against her closed labia, then opening so that it can press against her U-spot (*see* trigger points, page 153) and nudge against her vagina. However, the stimulation of choice with a vibrator is customarily her clitoris; she may need to start slowly if the stimulation is too much (choose a low speed or pad with a towel), then press in more firmly just behind the head. If he is working on her, he needs to know what to do at orgasm – some women need continuing stimulation, but for many the relentlessness of the vibrator against the swollen clitoris is too much; he will need to lift off slightly (or completely, then move in quickly to take her through with his tongue).

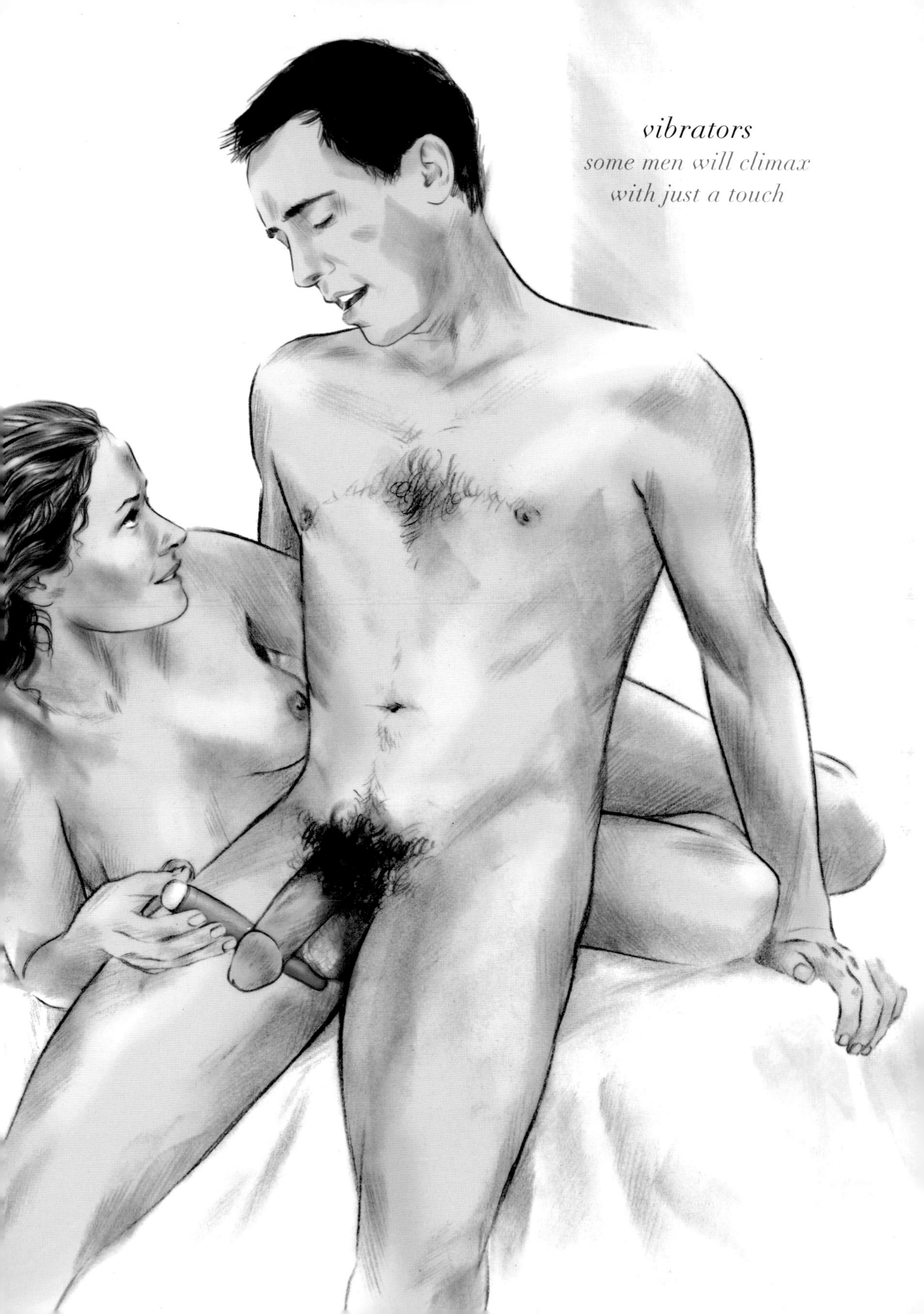

vibrators

some men will climax
with just a touch

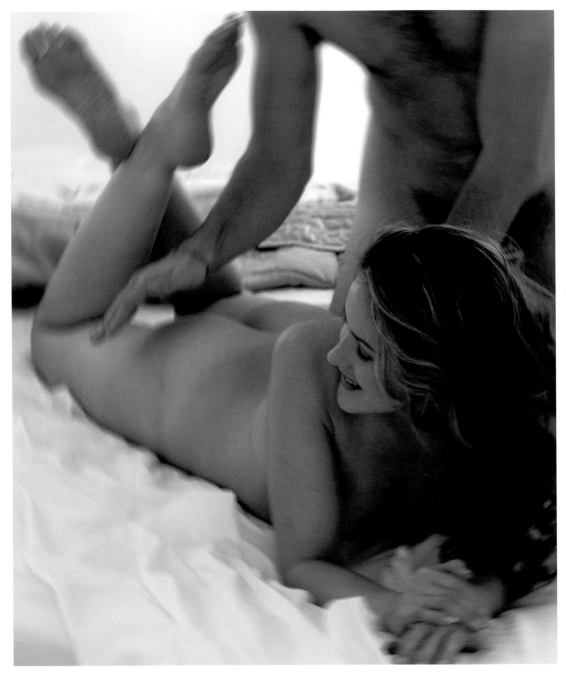

discipline
some people are wildly turned on by it

Beating is a turn-on that either works or doesn't. Quite apart from fantasists and talkers who are far more excited by the idea than the actual performance, some people are wildly turned on by it. For others, who have a real problem here, it may be necessary as a self-starter. Skin stimulation and the occasional spank at the right moment fit well into most people's repertoire. Most find that anything more is disappointing in proportion to the scale of the performance. If you are lovers and one of you wants to be on the receiving end, the other need not be scared that they will let out the beast in themselves by cooperating. If one of you wants to beat the other and he or she doesn't like it, or is turned off by the idea, that's non-negotiable – it surely doesn't need saying that all this should not be confused with abuse.

This is a clear case where if you can't communicate fantasies, you should not be lovers. Play it through a few times in words during straight intercourse (*see* birdsong at morning, pages 194–5). When you try it in practice, if it's the ritual that's the exciting part, make that big – don't be ashamed to ask for this, or give it: play matters. It can be a naughty child or a mistress-and-slave routine or whatever – if your partner's fantasy doesn't turn you on naturally, play it as a game and enjoy his or her response. If it's the physical sensation, rhythm and style apparently matter far more than force.

Start gently at around one blow in one or two seconds, not more. Allow the transformation effect to kick in (*see* pain, pages 264–5) before going full pelt, then gradually build up force until it's enough to make your subject want and not want you to stop. For two-way traffic, the result, plus struggling, should both look and feel sexy, not cruel. Never break the skin, and never beat neck, spine, or anywhere bony; stick to the buttocks or cover the whole surface – back, belly, and, if very lightly, breasts, penis (careful!), and vulva (put her on her back with her feet attached to the bedposts above her head, legs wide open; start on the buttocks, then give one light switch or two upon her thighs and vulva to finish her off). Or tie the victim's hands overhead to the shower nozzle and work them over under running water.

Traditional birch twigs are tricky to source, but sex shops offer whips and paddles that make a great noise but do no mischief; try them on yourself before using them on a partner and even then accept their judgment on what's hard and what's too hard. Or simply use your hand; a cupped palm will sound forceful yet create little pain, while an open flat palm will sting; apply an ice cube afterwards. Don't use bamboo – it cuts like a knife. Don't play this game with strangers, ever. Lovers have enough feedback not to let the most violent play go sour. And never mix purely erotic beating with real anger or bad temper (*see* hazards, pages 260–1). A game is a game is a game.

slow masturbation for her

The male-to-female version of the trick previously described (*see* slow masturbation for him, pages 269–71), usually possible only with a woman who is reliable in her orgasm, so she doesn't mind being slowed down or speeded up. The man has three points to concentrate on – mouth, breasts, and clitoris. He should stake her out, then start as she did, with the *coup de cassolette*

slow masturbation for her
make her scale another, still higher, range of peaks

(see pages 43–4), using armpit and glans, and then rub his hand over her *cassolette* and put it over her mouth, to play back her own perfume. He needs to gauge from her sounds and movements how heavy a touch on the clitoris she can stand. He can copy the spinning-out technique and excite her by postponement or he can simply push her as far and as fast as possible. If she is a responsive subject and not frightened of the whole business, the reaction will fully test his skill in securing her. He should kneel astride, but not sit on her, nor hold her down – she should be quite helpless anyway.

Finally, and in the case of experienced lovers this will be when she is semi-conscious, he will switch to a few moments of tongue work for lubrication, then vigorous intercourse and make her scale another, still higher, range of peaks, taking his own orgasm early on. He should know by the feel of her when to stop – this bears no relation to mewing and struggles, which reach a peak just short of climax. He should then untie her quickly, skillfully, and painlessly so that she comes back to earth lying quietly in his arms.

joy

From an evolutionary standpoint, sexual joy has a built-in sell-by date. Humans are hormonally programmed to lust until their genes have combined, then to support each other until the baby is born and self-sufficient, after which the genetic imperative becomes irrelevant. Nature sets no erotic targets for the postpartum couple unless it's to do it again. But surely more than this is possible. Humans are not just a collection of genes, not just a biological drive; we can feel, we can commit, we can love. Given that skill set, we can develop our potential in the sexual arena until we die.

The first step in this development is the determination never to accept mediocre. Sometimes you will both be tempted to settle for the comforting "do this, do that" sort of lovemaking that has always worked in the past and will do so again. This is fine on occasion or in the face of exhaustion, but serious lovers shouldn't be serving up that particular dish regularly. Challenge routines – as a matter of course and as an act of love – and challenge too the belief that you "shouldn't" or "can't" be more sexually daring. There is no such thing as too old, too staid, or too long-term a relationship.

In this regard, sex advisors recommend toys and dressing up; facile-sounding, but there's some truth in it. Anthropologist Helen Fisher points out that novelty triggers similar brain centers to passion, so by introducing new sexual variations, you replicate old romantic feelings. Acting on initial determination means being regularly willing to adapt foreplay, shift position, try games, set challenges, introduce accessories and props; always have somewhere new to go and something new to aim for. The Japanese had *shunga*, "pillow books" of sexual erotica and fantasy, for when inspiration faded; you could do worse than keep this very book in the bedside cabinet.

Above and beyond the props, however, you need to be willing to acknowledge that you want to do new and different things. The first, imprinting experience of each other's bodies may have been many years ago, and if you have changed over time – and all of us do – then your needs and tastes will have altered too. What turned you on two, five, or twenty years ago may no longer be what works. Admitting that to yourself and – much more scarily – admitting it to your partner takes courage, since it can stir up insecurities and resistance. But it's essential; acknowledging new and developing desires, then meeting them for oneself and one's partner is at the heart of all sexual development. Offering a menu of possibilities to fulfill those desires is at the heart of this book.

If there is one thing that will retain the joy of sex, it's continuing to say to your partner, "I really want you to . . . ," and continuing to respond to your partner with, "Yes . . ."

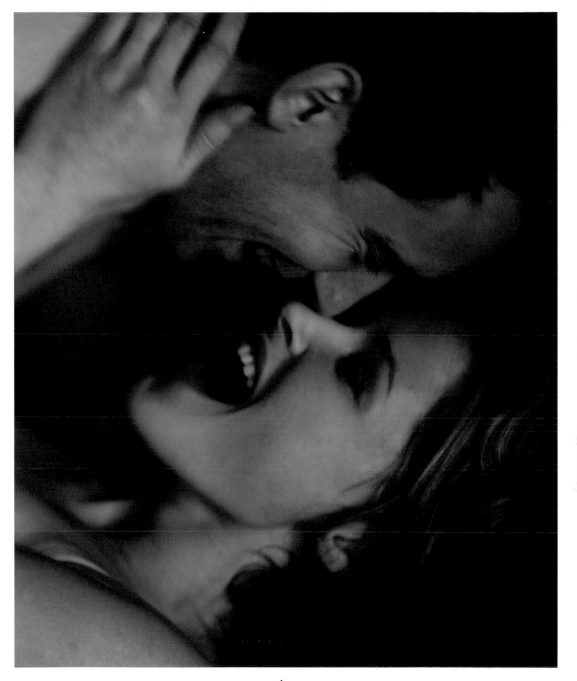

joy
always have somewhere new to go and something new to aim for

resources

birth control

National Women's Health Resource Center
1–877–986–9472
www.healthywomen.org
A nonprofit independent health information source for women.

Planned Parenthood Federation of America (PPFA)
1–800–230-PLAN
www.plannedparenthood.org
A women's health-care provider, educator, and advocate.

bisexual, gay, lesbian, and transsexual

The Advocate Guide to Gay Men's Health and Wellness, by Frank Spinelli, M.D. (New York: Alyson Books, 2008).
A comprehensive medical guide for gay men by New York City's "hottest gay doctor."

Anal Pleasure & Health: A Guide for Men and Women, by Jack Morin (San Francisco: Down There Press, 1998).
Though not gay specific, this guide includes gay-related information on having a healthy sex life.

CenterLink (formerly The National Association of Lesbian, Gay, Bisexual and Transgender Community Centers)
www.lgbtcenters.org
A member-based coalition to support the development of strong, sustainable LGBT community centers.

Fenway Guide to Lesbian, Gay, Bisexual & Transgender Health, Harvey J. Makadon, Kenneth H. Mayer, Jennifer Potter, and Hilary Goldhammer, editors (Philadelphia: American College of Physicians, 2007).
Guidance, practical guidelines, and discussions of clinical issues pertinent to the LGBT patient and community.

Gay.com
www.gay.com
An online community for gay individuals.

Gay and Lesbian Medical Association
www.glma.org
The world's largest and oldest association of lesbian, gay, bisexual, and transgender health-care professionals.

GLBT National Health Center
1–888-THE-GLNH (national hotline)
1–888–246-PRIDE (national youth talk line)
www.glnh.org
Provides free and confidential telephone and e-mail peer counseling, information, and local resources for GLBT and questioning individuals.

The Gay Men's Health Crisis
www.gmhc.org
GMHC offers an array of programs and services to thousands of men, women, and children every year.

The Network/La Red
1–617–742–4911
www.thenetworklared.org
A group that works to end abuse in lesbian, bisexual women's, and transgender communities.

cancers–female sexual

I Am Not Breast Cancer: Women Talk Openly About Love and Sex, Hair Loss and Weight Gain, Mothers and Daughters, and Being a Woman with Breast Cancer, by Ruth Peltason (New York: William Morrow, 2008).
Entries from eight hundred women around the world offer comfort, strength, and hope.

National Cervical Cancer Coalition
www.nccc online.org
A coalition battling cervical cancer and HPV-related issues.

National Ovarian Cancer Coalition
www.ovarian.org
A group dedicated to offering education, support, and hope for patients and to raising awareness of ovarian cancer across the country.

Y-ME National Breast Cancer Organization
1–800–221–2141
www.y-me.org
Support, information, and resources for women battling breast cancer.

cancers–male sexual

Surviving Prostate Cancer: What You Need to Know to Make Informed Decisions, by E. Fuller Torrey (New Haven, Conn.: Yale University Press Health & Wellness, 2008).
A doctor's account of battling and surviving prostate cancer, complete with personal experience and factual material.

Testicular Cancer Information & Support
www.tc-cancer.com
Education and support for patients with testicular cancer and their families.

eating disorders

National Eating Disorders Association
800.931.2237
www.edap.org
The largest nonprofit organization in the United States working to prevent eating disorders and provide treatment referrals to those suffering from eating disorders and body-image and weight issues.

National Health Information Center
www.health.gov/nhic
NHIC offers a nationwide referral service and produces directories and resource guides.

infertility

National Infertility Network Exchange
www.nine-infertility.org
A national nonprofit organization for persons and couples with impaired fertility, and the professionals that serve them.

National Women's Health Information Center
www.4women.gov
Information and resources on women's health.

support

If a lack of joy in sex is an occasional, minor issue, there are helpful suggestions throughout the book. If it's a serious issue, you should look further afield.

In our society there are still taboos about doing that; a problem may feel too small, too big, or too embarrassing to seek help in addressing. You should still do so – not just because there are far fewer taboos now but also because there is far more available help. Over the past fifty years, medical and counseling treatments have improved beyond all recognition; by treating a physical condition, resolving a past trauma, increasing knowledge, improving communication, changing inaccurate attitudes, or rebuilding a failing relationship, there is a very good chance of a solution.

Do both partners of a couple have to seek help? Ideally, but not necessarily; if one alone is helped, that may well impact on the other. But it is loving good practice, when it comes to sexual problems just as much as sex itself, to hold a partner's hand. Problem-solve together if you can – whether when reading a self-help book or seeing a counselor.

Here are some general guidelines on finding help; accessibility will vary from country to country and culture to culture.

- **Self-help books** Details of favorites follow; *see* resources, pages 278–81. If you are choosing your own, avoid ones that make extravagant claims, those written by authors with affiliations to commercial enterprises, and those that sound as if they will perform miracles; they won't. A textbook on a sexual problem, or a book written by an academic, may be drier than a popularization but is likely to be more accurate.

- **Organizations** For most problems, there are corresponding national or international organizations; the best offer information, guidelines, a telephone help line, chat rooms for sufferer support, networking opportunities, advisory boards to which you can write and get personalized answers, lists of practitioners, even training courses and conferences.

  Almost all reputable ones are now available on the Internet; *see* resources, pages 278–81, for details. For local options, search on the name of the problem plus key words such as "symptoms . . . treatments." The upside of the Web means that this will bring you instant access to all the best sites; the downside is that these may well be intermingled with the worst. To sort the sheep from the goats, remember that those affiliated to charitable rather than product-selling organizations will be more useful, as will websites for national or group schemes rather than individual practitioners.

- **Help lines** Many organizations also run help lines, and additionally there are help lines not affiliated to other organizational services. Both offer anonymous and immediate advice. Good ones will be informed about sexual problems, and happy to give information and offer short-term emotional support. However, don't expect medical diagnosis, or in-depth or long-term counseling. It will help, before phoning, to make a list of your symptoms or problems and any previous treatment you have had or any action you have taken.

- **Heath and medical professions** Seeing your own general practitioner is an essential first step in checking out any sexual problem, not only because the problem itself may be due to a health condition or a side effect of its treatment, but also because more difficulties than before are now helped by medical solutions. If the clinician you consult is hostile or embarrassed, change clinicians; as with all services, shop around.

- **Face-to-face support** If you have ruled out medical issues, or if you suspect that what underpins your problems is a personal hang-up or a relationship difficulty, see a counselor. Ways of tracking such down will vary, but the relevant national organization for each specific problem will often have a list of therapists, as may your general practitioner.

  It's best to phone the counselor first to check out basic issues, such as where they live and how much they charge. Then arrange an exploratory visit; once there, ask further questions regarding their experience and their working methods, and assess whether you and they get along. Training and qualifications are important, but have been proved to be less crucial for treatment success than experience and rapport with you, the client.

- **Exercises** Many counselors will ask you not only to discuss problems but also to talk through sexual issues or practice sexual techniques at home. In particular, they may ask you to masturbate alone or together; to practice "sensate focus," a way of relearning how to touch and be touched; to experiment with ways of managing his erection and her orgasm. Neither counselors nor physicians, however, should ever ask you to be sexual with them or in front of them, or to undress without a chaperone present. Practicing techniques is an integral part of much sexual counseling, but you should do this only so far and so fast as you are comfortable.

For all the above, from books to experts, the key is whether you feel at ease with them. If not, however qualified, lauded, or credible your sources of help, look elsewhere.

acknowledgments

Firstly, deepest thanks to Nick Comfort for his ongoing support and encouragement as I reinvented his father's book. Equal thanks also to all the friends and colleagues who helped make that reinvention happen, particularly to: Barbara Levy for her continuing professional and personal backing; Joy Haughton for her bright intelligence, ideas, and stamina; Laura Bates for her delightful attitude to work and particular talent in brainstorming; Clare Button for her utterly tireless ability to sort out tiny pieces of information; Colin Marsh for energetically balancing books; Sara Nazzerzadeh for insightful cross-cultural expertise; and all the great people at Mitchell Beazley for bringing everything to a triumphant fruition. Last but by no means least, thanks to the Shaft of Darkness Club for their ability to answer the most esoteric of questions.

Susan Quilliam

index

Figures in *italics* indicate captions.